# Advance Directives, Durable Power of Attorney, Wills, and Other Legal Considerations

*Laura Town and Karen Hoffman*

Omega Press
Zionsville, IN 46077
© 2024 Omega Press

ISBN-13: 978-1-943414-38-3

While we have made every attempt to ensure that the information contained in this book has been obtained from reliable sources, Laura Town, Karen Hoffman, and Omega Press are not responsible for any errors or omissions or for the results obtained from the use of this information. The information is provided "as is" without warranty of any kind. The information available in this book is for informational purposes only and not for the purpose of providing legal, financial, or healthcare advice. You should contact your attorney, financial planner, or physician to obtain advice with respect to any particular issue or problem. In addition, Laura Town, Karen Hoffman, and Omega Press do not endorse any products mentioned in this book, nor do they assume any responsibility for the interpretation or application of any information originating from such content.

**Production Credits:**
Authors: Laura Town and Karen Hoffman
Publisher: Omega Press
Photos: All credited images used under license from Shutterstock.com

**Social media connections:**
Laura Town
LinkedIn: https://www.linkedin.com/in/lauratown

Karen Hoffman
LinkedIn: https://www.linkedin.com/in/karen-hoffman-91502b62/

# Omega Press Books

### *How to Save Money on Healthcare*

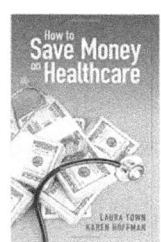

- People in the United States have over $220 billion in medical debt
- 20% of Americans have some type of medical debt
- Over 60% of bankruptcies are related to medical debt
- 25% of adults have skipped or postponed getting needed health care because of the cost
- About half of adults would be unable to pay unexpected medical expenses over $500
- Audiobook, ebook, and paperback available on Amazon

## *Long-Term Care Insurance, Power of Attorney, Wealth Management, and Other First Steps*

- Getting long-term care insurance earlier is better. Only 20% of people age 50-59 were declined for long-term care insurance, but almost 50% of people age 70-74 were declined.
- Two-thirds of Americans do not have an estate plan, and more than half of people don't know where their parents store their estate planning documents.
- Of those who do have an estate plan, one-third did not include power of attorney documents.
- Audiobook and ebook available on Amazon

---

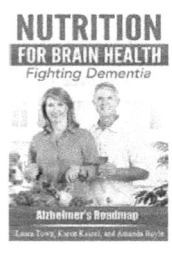

## *Nutrition for Brain Health: Fighting Dementia*

- A Seniorlink (www.seniorlink.com) 50 Essential Read for Anyone Coping with Alzheimer's Disease
- Audiobook, ebook, and paperback available wherever books are sold

# CONTENTS

**Introduction**..................................................1
  *Checklist: Legal documents needed for individuals with Alzheimer's disease*........................... 2

**Chapter 1: Elder Law Attorneys** ...................3
  *Checklist: How to find a good elder law attorney* ............. 4
  *Checklist: How to prepare for your elder law attorney appointment*....................... 7
  *Checklist: Topics to discuss with your elder law attorney* .. 9
  *Checklist: Reasons to review legal documents*................... 11

**Chapter 2: Discussing Legal Documents**................... 13
  *Checklist: How to discuss legal documents with your loved one*.............................. 14

**Chapter 3: Legal Documents for Healthcare** ............ 19
  DURABLE POWER OF ATTORNEY FOR HEALTHCARE 19
  *Checklist: Basics about a durable power of attorney for healthcare*..................... 19
  *Checklist: Responsibilities of the principal.* ..................... 21
  *Checklist: Characteristics of a good healthcare agent*........ 23
  *Checklist: Responsibilities of a healthcare agent* .............. 25
  ADVANCE DIRECTIVES....................................... 30
  Living Will.................................................. 31
  *Checklist: Basics about a living will* ............................... 31
  *Checklist: Medical treatments that may be covered in a*

*living will* ........................................................................ 33

   *Checklist: Responsibilities of the principal* ...................... 34

   *Checklist: Situations to consider when deciding about life-prolonging medical procedures* ........................................... 35

Do Not Resuscitate and Do Not Intubate ................ 36

   *Checklist: Basics about DNR and DNI orders* ............. 37

   *Checklist: When should my loved one have a DNR order?* ............................................................................................. 39

   *Checklist: When should my loved one NOT have a DNR order?* ........................................................................... 40

Clinically Administered Nutrition and Hydration .... 40

   *Checklist: Basics about clinically administered nutrition and hydration* ....................................................................... 41

Organ, Tissue, and Body Donation ............................ 42

   *Checklist: Basics about organ, tissue, and body donation* 43

Other Directives ............................................................ 44

   *Checklist: Basics about less-common medical directives* .... 44

PHYSICIAN ORDERS FOR LIFE-SUSTAINING TREATMENT (POLST) ....................................................... 47

## Chapter 4: Legal Documents for Finances ............... 49

DURABLE POWER OF ATTORNEY FOR FINANCES ....... 49

   *Checklist: Basics about a durable power of attorney for finances* ......................................................................... 50

   *Checklist: Responsibilities of the principal* ...................... 51

   *Checklist: Characteristics of a good attorney-in-fact* ......... 52

   *Checklist: Responsibilities of an attorney-in-fact* ............... 53

LAST WILL AND TESTAMENT .......................................... 55

*Checklist: Basics about a last will and testament............ 56*
*Checklist: Responsibilities of the testator......................... 58*
*Checklist: Items commonly listed in the will..................... 59*
*Checklist: Characteristics of a good executor of the will... 63*
*Checklist: Responsibilities of an executor of the will......... 64*
TRUSTS ................................................................................ 65
*Checklist: Terms related to trusts ..................................... 65*
*Checklist: Types of trusts ................................................. 66*
*Checklist: What to put in a trust...................................... 68*
*Checklist: How do I know if my loved one needs a trust? 69*
*Checklist: How do I help my loved one create a trust?..... 70*
*Checklist: Characteristics of a good trustee...................... 71*
*Checklist: Responsibilities of a trustee.............................. 72*

## Chapter 5: Other Legal Documents ........................ 71
POWER OF ATTORNEY...................................................... 71
General Power of Attorney............................................ 71
Springing Power of Attorney........................................ 72
HEALTHCARE PROXY....................................................... 72
CONSERVATORSHIP/GUARDIANSHIP............................ 72
GUARDIANSHIP OF MINOR CHILDREN ......................... 74
*Checklist: Things to consider when choosing a good guardian for children......................................................................... 75*
ADMINISTRATOR.............................................................. 76
GOVERNMENT BENEFITS ................................................ 76
SOCIAL MEDIA WILL........................................................ 77

 Ethical Will .................................................................. 78

## Chapter 6: Dealing with Conflict ............................... 79
 *Checklist: Common causes of conflict* .............................. *79*
 *Checklist: Strategies to prevent or resolve conflict* ............. *81*

## Conclusion .................................................................. 84

## About the Authors ..................................................... 85
 Laura Town ................................................................... 85
 Karen Hoffman ............................................................. 86
 A Note from the Authors ........................................... 87
 Additional Titles from Laura Town and Karen Hoffman ........................................................................ 88

## Resources .................................................................... 89

## Reference List ............................................................. 95

# Introduction

A diagnosis of Alzheimer's disease can be devastating to you and your loved one. All individuals with Alzheimer's disease eventually become unable to make good decisions about their healthcare and finances. Therefore, having written legal documents in place that help you know the wishes of your loved one relieves some of the burden of making hard choices about medical care and helps avoid conflict between family and friends over possessions and healthcare decisions.

With my (Laura's) dad's disease journey, we endured a lot of drama. He got lost in France, he was convinced that Nigerians were going to kidnap him, and he hitchhiked. I was fortunate, however, that he was docile and agreeable when I decided to take control over his financial and legal affairs. I think he was at the point where he knew he needed that. One of my childhood friends, Amy, had a completely different experience. Her dad refused to allow Amy to even know where the checkbook was, much less sign off on any legal or financial papers that would give her any control.

Like Amy, your loved one may resent you for asking them to turn over legal control of their finances or healthcare to you or another trusted individual. This resentment is part of the disease process, and it is something you will have to make peace with. Unfortunately, nothing is easy about helping a loved one endure Alzheimer's disease. You can only do the best you can for your loved one and accept the hurt feelings that result, knowing that your loved one's responses are caused by the disease and their fear over losing their independence.

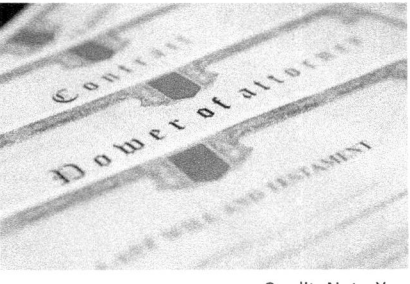

Credit: NotarYes

Because your loved one must be legally competent to sign legal documents pertaining to healthcare and finances, you should help your loved one prepare these legal documents as soon as possible. The checklist below provides a list of legal documents that your loved one should prepare now before they are no longer able to share their wishes with you. These documents will ensure that your loved one's wishes are being met even if they can no longer make their preferences known. This book describes these and other documents, what you need in order to prepare each document, and the responsibilities of individuals named in the documents.

*Checklist: Legal documents needed for individuals with Alzheimer's disease*

**Recommended**

- ☐ Durable Power of Attorney for Healthcare
- ☐ Durable Power of Attorney for Finances
- ☐ Living Will
- ☐ Last Will and Testament

**Optional**

- ☐ Living Trust
- ☐ Do Not Resuscitate (DNR) Order
- ☐ Do Not Intubate (DNI) Order

# Chapter 1:
# Elder Law Attorneys

Legal documents can be confusing, and different states have different requirements and different terminology for legal documents pertaining to healthcare and finances. Therefore, searching for a trusted elder law attorney is a good starting point for many families or friends with a loved one who was recently diagnosed with Alzheimer's disease.

Elder law attorneys specialize in legal documents related to elderly care, including options for healthcare, distribution of possessions, and receipt of Medicare or Medicaid services. Elder law attorneys understand your state's requirements for documents such as living wills and Do Not Resuscitate orders. They also know the proper procedures for appointing a power of attorney for your loved one.

If your loved one does not already have legal documents in place, finding a good elder law attorney should be done as quickly as possible after your loved one's diagnosis. It is important for your loved one to be able to make decisions about legal matters while they can still understand and give consent to the documents; this is called "legal capacity" or "competency." Once your loved one's mental abilities begin to decline, they are no longer qualified to sign legal documents, and it will be easier for family members to contest the documents if they don't agree with the stipulations in the documents.

I will admit it, I'm cheap. In my dad's case, I was hoping that I could prepare legal documents on the Internet or with the use of legal software. However, when I met with the elder law attorney we chose, she brought up scenarios that I had not contemplated. She also told us ways we could effectively protect Dad's assets and handle the taxes that I did not know about. Even though I spent $250 per hour for the attorney, I was relieved. The legal advice I received

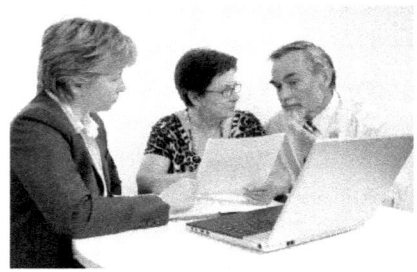
Credit: Alexander Raths

saved me more in the long run than if I'd relied on a software program that could not possibly take into account my particular circumstances. Keep in mind that attorney fees may differ in different geographic locations. Different states, cities, or countries will have different standards for attorney fees and other costs associated with creating legal documents.

Having a good elder law attorney can ease some stress, but how do you go about finding the right attorney for your needs? The following checklist provides some questions to ask when searching for an elder law attorney.

## *Checklist: How to find a good elder law attorney*

- ☐ Does this attorney live in my area? You can find attorneys in your area by searching online or in the phone book for elder law attorneys. The national registry for elder law attorneys at https://www.naela.org can also help.

- ☐ Does this attorney understand my state's requirements for legal documents?

- ☐ Does this attorney handle all the legal documents I need to make? For example, do they understand estate law, trust law, healthcare decision making, and senior housing options?

- ☐ Does this attorney understand Medicare and Medicaid requirements, and are they able to make suggestions and handle paperwork regarding qualifications for Medicare and Medicaid?

- ☐ How long has this attorney practiced elder law?

- ☐ What percentage of this attorney's practice focuses on elder law?
- ☐ Is this attorney a Certified Elder Law Attorney?
- ☐ Is this attorney active in professional and community organizations?
- ☐ Is there a fee for the first consultation? If so, what is it?
- ☐ How does this attorney charge fees? By the hour? By the document? What is the attorney's hourly or per document rate? Will my loved one be able to afford these fees?
- ☐ How frequently does this attorney bill my loved one? Weekly? Monthly? Upon completion of work?
- ☐ Does this attorney charge for out-of-pocket expenses such as copies, postage fees, etc.?
- ☐ Does this attorney charge for over-the-phone consultations or questions?
- ☐ How frequently does this attorney recommend reviewing legal documents to make sure they are up to date? What is the fee for this service?
- ☐ Will this attorney charge fees if my loved one wants to make any changes to their documents later? If so, what are these fees?
- ☐ How will my loved one's documents be protected from change if they are no longer competent to make changes? Will the attorney refuse to make changes to legal documents if someone else (not a legal surrogate) brings in the loved one to make changes?
- ☐ Will this attorney require a retainer? (A retainer is money paid to the attorney before work starts, and the attorney pays themselves from these funds.)

- How long is a typical waiting period for getting an appointment with this attorney?
- Is this attorney able to handle decision-making responsibilities in my absence?
- Is this attorney willing to be an executor or administrator of my loved one's estate if I need this service?
- Will this attorney provide advice on how to "spend down" my loved one's assets to help qualify for Medicaid, if I decide to do this?
- Is this attorney willing to mediate between family members in the event of family disagreements? Or do they have a mediator that they recommend?
- Is this attorney familiar with local long-term care facilities and the practices they follow in accepting or denying patients?
- Do I know anyone who has used this attorney? If so, do they recommend this attorney?
- Are there any online reviews about this attorney or law firm? If so, are they generally positive or negative reviews?

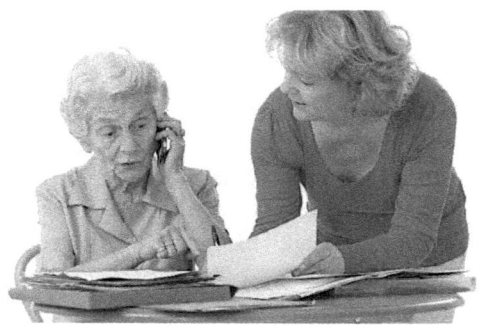

Credit: JPC-PROD

Once you or your loved one has contacted several elder law attorneys and selected the one that is the best fit for your loved one's needs, how should you prepare for that first appointment? The following checklist details the information you will need to gather before your first appointment with an elder law attorney. You may want to contact your elder law attorney to determine what information they will need to complete your loved one's legal documents. Different documents may require different information.

## *Checklist: How to prepare for your elder law attorney appointment*

- ☐ Gather information about your loved one's personal records, including legal name; Social Security number; place and date of birth; locations of legal documents such as birth certificates and marriage certificates; and education, employment, and military records.

- ☐ Gather information about your loved one's medical condition, including diagnosis, current stage of illness, and ability to care for themself.

- ☐ Determine the overall financial needs and resources of your loved one. Will your loved one have enough in savings and retirement income to cover their needs? Will your loved one qualify for federal or state financial assistance?

- ☐ Gather documents related to your loved one's bank accounts, including checking accounts, savings accounts, and certificates of deposit.

- ☐ Gather documents related to your loved one's recent federal and state tax returns.

- ☐ Gather documents related to your loved one's sources of income, such as Social Security, disability, pensions, retirement accounts, veteran benefits, investments, rental property, and other income.

- Gather documents related to your loved one's investments, including stocks, bonds, mutual funds, and other investments.
- Gather documents related to your loved one's property, including real estate, vehicles, and personal possessions, especially valuable possessions such as jewelry. Also determine if your loved one has a safe deposit box and what the box contains.
- Gather documents related to your loved one's insurance policies, including health insurance, home insurance, car insurance, long-term care insurance, life insurance, Medicare, Medicaid, and any other insurance policy.
- Gather legal documents related to healthcare and possessions, such as a power of attorney, living will, trusts, or last will and testament.
- Gather information regarding your loved one's debt, including mortgages, loans, unpaid bills, credit cards, and other debt. If your loved one owns a business that has debt and your loved one is personally responsible for that debt, that information should be gathered as well.
- Gather documents related to your loved one's admission to a healthcare facility.
- Find out if your loved one has legal responsibility for another individual, such as a spouse or an adult child with disabilities. What are the needs of this individual?

- ☐ Determine the likelihood that your loved one will need full-time care assistance, either at home or in a long-term care facility. You may need to discuss this with your loved one's physician and other trusted individuals who may help with your loved one's care.
- ☐ Discuss the likelihood of you and other primary caregivers becoming disabled and/or unable to care for your loved one.
- ☐ Determine who will care for your loved one if you are unable to do so. This individual should be listed in legal documents as a successor as appropriate.
- ☐ Gather information about all involved parties, including descendants, spouses, other family members, caregivers, financial planners, family attorneys, accountants, and others. You should be able to provide contact information for each individual.
- ☐ Ask the attorney if you need to bring other documents or information to the appointment, such as specific forms of identification.

Once you and your loved one have selected an elder law attorney and gathered the information you need for your first appointment, you must decide what to discuss during your appointment. The following checklist reviews important discussion topics.

## *Checklist: Topics to discuss with your elder law attorney*

- ☐ Discuss options for healthcare, including durable power of attorney for healthcare, living wills, Do Not Resuscitate (DNR) orders, and Do Not Intubate (DNI) orders.

- ☐ Discuss options for possessions, including durable power of attorney for finances, last will and testament, and living trusts.
- ☐ Discuss options for guardianship of minor children and adult children with disabilities, which should be included in guardianship documents (transfer guardianship before death) as well as in the last will and testament (transfer guardianship after death).
- ☐ Discuss options for financing care, including personal funds, investment income, Medicare, Medicaid, insurance, veteran's benefits, and Social Security.
- ☐ Discuss options for living arrangements, including long-term care or in-home care.

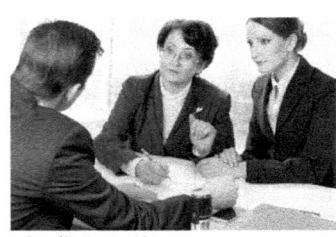

Credit: NotarYes

Once you have legal documents in place, you should review documents periodically to ensure that they still reflect your loved one's current wishes. This review should happen as frequently as needed while your loved one is still legally competent to make changes to each document. The following checklist provides some important reasons to review legal documents. Note that although some of the reasons are listed under a specific document, they may apply to more than one document. In addition, the documents should be reviewed, but they do not *have* to be changed unless your loved one deems it necessary.

## *Checklist: Reasons to review legal documents*

### Power of attorney

- ☐ Your loved one is no longer legally qualified to be a power of attorney (also applies to executor of the will and trustees).
- ☐ The person listed as the power of attorney is no longer capable or willing to manage financial or healthcare decisions (also applies to executor of the will and trustees). This may happen if family tensions, health, or other circumstances cause too much stress for the individual.
- ☐ The person listed as the power of attorney consistently goes against your loved one's wishes or abuses their power.
- ☐ The person listed as the power of attorney no longer lives in close proximity to your loved one (either because they moved or because your loved one moved).

### Living will and advance directives

- ☐ Your loved one has a change in health or mental state.
- ☐ Your loved one's living arrangements change.
- ☐ Your loved one changes their mind about contents of the legal document (applies to all legal documents).

### Last will and testament and living trust

- ☐ Your loved one retires.
- ☐ Your loved one moves to a different state.

- ☐ There is a birth, adoption, or death in the family.
- ☐ There is a marriage or divorce in the family.
- ☐ There is a falling out or reconciliation between your loved one and another family member or friend.
- ☐ A minor child who is under your loved one's guardianship turns 18.
- ☐ Beneficiaries reach a milestone age or personal situation as stated by the will or trust (e.g., items in a trust may transfer to an individual at the age of 25, when they get married, and so on).
- ☐ Beneficiaries are added to or removed from accounts.
- ☐ Property or investments are bought or sold.
- ☐ Sources of income or debt change.
- ☐ Tax laws change.
- ☐ There is a substantial increase or decrease in your loved one's estate.
- ☐ There is a substantial change to a business owned by your loved one.
- ☐ A family member states a preference for inheriting a specific item, as long as the rest of the family is in agreement.
- ☐ A charity that interests your loved one opens, closes, or has a change in needs that your loved one wants to support.

# Chapter 2:
# Discussing Legal Documents

Creating legal documents as soon as possible, either before or after diagnosis, is the best way to ensure that your loved one's wishes are followed when they become mentally incompetent or pass away. In order for your loved one to sign legal documents, they must be mentally competent, able to make rational decisions, and able to understand the contents of the documents and the legal ramifications of signing the documents. For individuals with dementia such as Alzheimer's disease, the earlier these documents are signed in the course of the disease, the more likely it is that the documents will stand firm in a court of law.

If your loved one was recently diagnosed with Alzheimer's disease and they do not have the recommended legal documents in place, you need to encourage them to start thinking about and creating these documents. Some individuals may feel that this is the beginning of their loss of independence, and the realization that they can no longer be completely independent may be a source of contention. People react differently to these types of requests from loved ones.

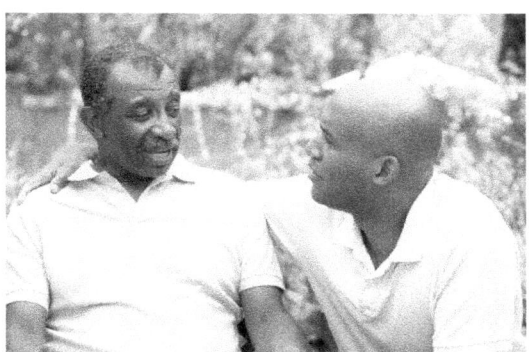

Credit: Monkey Business Images

In my friend Amy's case, her father was giving money away to scam artists and making questionable purchases on a limited income. Amy knew that she had to act soon or her parents would be in a worse position. Because her father refused to discuss legal documents with her, Amy asked her father's friends to convince her dad to relinquish control.

Amy needed a unique approach when talking to her father about legal documents. You may also find that you need to try several approaches before one works. The following checklist provides some ideas for how to start the discussion about legal documents with your loved one. Some of these ideas may be more appropriate for you and your loved one than others, so use the ones that seem most natural for you. Keep in mind that you may have to take control of your loved one's finances and legal matters against their wishes for their own good, perhaps even going to court to officially have them declared legally incompetent if that is what it takes.

## *Checklist: How to discuss legal documents with your loved one*

- ☐ Ask permission to talk about end-of-life issues because many people avoid this topic.
- ☐ Ask your loved one if they have considered what will happen to them and their possessions if they become incapacitated or die.
- ☐ Tell your loved one that you are in the process of making these legal documents for yourself, and encourage them to take steps to make these legal documents for themself.
- ☐ Start with a story of someone else's experience of how they wished they would have had legal documents in place or they were thankful that they had such documents.

- ☐ Ask a close friend of your loved one or your loved one's minister to encourage them to get their affairs in order.

- ☐ Take notice of opportunities to open the conversation, such as the death of a loved one, a news story, medical checkups, family gatherings, movies, sermons, and others. Follow through with the conversation about legal documents as opportunities appear.

- ☐ If you are the spouse, ask your loved one to discuss legal matters with you so you can make decisions together now rather than having to make them alone later.

- ☐ If you are the adult child, ask your parents and siblings to hold a family meeting (immediate family only) to discuss important legal matters. Turn it into a family project in which everyone creates their own legal documents.

- ☐ Make an "appointment" to discuss legal matters. Select an appropriate time and place for the discussion; a private place is usually best. Keep the discussion light and make an event of it.

- ☐ Mention to your loved one that talking about this earlier and more frequently will help you ensure that their wishes are being met in the future because you and other caregivers will understand what they would have chosen for themself.

- ☐ Tell your loved one that having the discussion now will save a lot of pain and anxiety for caregivers later.

- ☐ Mention that your loved one's attorney or physician mentioned that it would be helpful to create legal documents related to finances and healthcare.

- ☐ Encourage your loved one to speak with their physician about medical options at the end of life so they understand the options they want to list in their legal documents.

- ☐ Start discussions early. It is more comfortable to talk about these topics when it is a hypothetical future issue rather than a current, looming one. For individuals with Alzheimer's disease, waiting too long could mean that they are no longer legally competent to make legal documents.

- ☐ Don't be surprised if you encounter resistance the first time you try. Don't be discouraged or force the issue. Come back to the discussion later when an opening presents itself.

- ☐ Allow your loved one to set the pace of the conversation.

- ☐ Make sure you are a good listener during the conversation. Listen for clues about your loved one's wishes and don't turn it into a debate.

- ☐ Be caring and supportive, and don't be selfish or demanding.

- ☐ If your loved one is already making poor financial choices and refuses to sign legal documents, you may need to take them to court to have them declared legally incompetent in order to have a conservator or guardian appointed for them.

- ☐ If your loved one already has legal documents in place, ask them to review the documents to make sure they still reflect their wishes in light of their new diagnosis.

- ☐ Make sure your loved one knows you want to have this discussion because you care about them.

Starting the discussion about legal documents is perhaps the most uncomfortable part of the entire process. Once your loved one has accepted the fact that legal documents need to be created, the process of making the documents can be tedious but also rewarding and comforting. The most important documents to create are the durable power of attorney for healthcare and durable power of attorney for finances. Once these documents are in place, you and your loved one can focus on creating a living will and other advance directives as well as creating a last will and testament and living trust, if desired.

# Chapter 3:
# Legal Documents for Healthcare

Your loved one's need for good healthcare will grow as they progress through Alzheimer's disease. However, at some point in the course of the disease, your loved one will be unable to make their own healthcare choices, either because they cannot understand their medical choices, they cannot rationally make a decision, or they are unable to communicate their wishes. Therefore, having legal documents related to their healthcare wishes is vital to them receiving the care they would have chosen for themself. Legal documents related to healthcare include a durable power of attorney for healthcare, living will, and other advance directives.

## Durable Power of Attorney for Healthcare

A durable power of attorney for healthcare is created to name a single individual or group of individuals who will be allowed to make healthcare decisions for your loved one. A durable power of attorney for healthcare is called "durable" because it is active both before and after the principal is declared mentally incompetent. Choosing a good healthcare agent is one of the most important legal decisions your loved one will make. See the following checklists for important aspects to consider when creating a durable power of attorney for healthcare.

*Checklist: Basics about a durable power of attorney for healthcare*

- ☐ The durable power of attorney for healthcare document may also be called a healthcare power of attorney, medical power of attorney, appointment of a healthcare agent, or healthcare proxy.

- The individual creating the durable power of attorney for healthcare is called the principal. In this book, your loved one with Alzheimer's disease is assumed to be the principal.
- The individual named to make healthcare decisions for the principal is called the healthcare agent. They may also be called a surrogate, attorney-in-fact, healthcare representative, or healthcare proxy.
- The healthcare agent is only allowed to make medical decisions, not financial decisions, for your loved one.
- The durable power of attorney for healthcare is valid for both temporary (e.g., after an accident) and permanent (e.g., late-stage Alzheimer's disease) incapacitation.
- Although the durable power of attorney for healthcare is valid as soon as it is signed, physicians usually do not take advice from the healthcare agent as long as the principal is capable of making decisions.
- The durable power of attorney for healthcare can be revoked or changed at any time as long as your loved one is still legally competent.

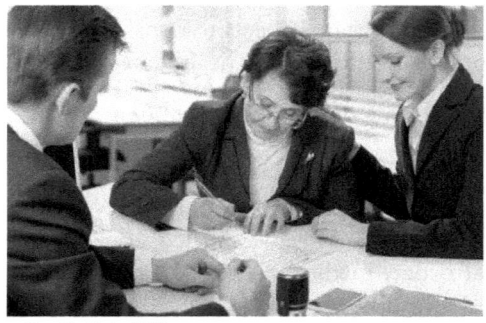

Credit: NotarYES

- Your loved one should include a HIPAA release in the durable power of attorney for healthcare so that the healthcare agent can access your loved one's medical records.
- A major benefit to having a healthcare agent, instead of having only a living will, is that the healthcare agent can make all healthcare decisions in real time based on current information, whereas the living will is designed for a limited number of hypothetical situations. For this reason, some attorneys recommend against creating a living will and instead having only a healthcare agent, assuming the healthcare agent is trustworthy.
- If your loved one becomes incapacitated and does not have a healthcare agent, they will either be appointed a healthcare proxy by a physician (a short-term solution) or will need to have a guardian appointed by the court (a long-term solution).

## *Checklist: Responsibilities of the principal.*

- Determine whether any state laws restrict the choice of healthcare agent. For example, does the healthcare agent have to be a resident of the same state as your loved one?
- Choose a healthcare agent based on desired characteristics of a healthcare agent. Make sure the chosen agent is willing to accept this responsibility. Some states require that only one healthcare agent has power at a time, but some allow multiple agents.
- If more than one healthcare agent is chosen to act at the same time, all agents must be present and agree on medical actions before medical personnel will act on the decisions. This makes it complicated

for physicians to act, especially if the agents do not agree.

- ☐ Choose an alternative healthcare agent if the original healthcare agent is unavailable or is unwilling to serve.
- ☐ Stipulate any restrictions on the healthcare agent, such as when the agent can make decisions (e.g., after diagnosis of a terminal illness, when the principal is permanently unconscious, etc.).
- ☐ Name any individuals who should not have any role in making healthcare decisions. This may be an estranged family member or in-laws.
- ☐ Create and sign the durable power of attorney for healthcare document. If your loved one spends significant time in more than one state, a durable power of attorney for healthcare document should be created for each state.
- ☐ Distribute copies of the durable power of attorney for healthcare to regular healthcare providers, the local hospital, the healthcare agent and alternative healthcare agent, and close family members.
- ☐ Keep a copy of the durable power of attorney document in an easily accessible place at home, and tell the healthcare agent and close family members where to find the document.
- ☐ Discuss responsibilities of the healthcare agent and any advance directives with the chosen agent(s).
- ☐ Discuss with the healthcare agent any values and beliefs that would affect healthcare decisions. Examples are religious beliefs that would dictate refusal of medical treatments, values that give your loved one's life meaning (family, career,

independence, etc.), concerns about death or dying, and financial concerns.
- ☐ Tell family members who the chosen healthcare agent is and why they were chosen.
- ☐ If one healthcare agent becomes unwilling or unable to serve, or if your loved one wishes to revoke the agent's power, your loved one will need to create a new document and destroy all old documents.

## *Checklist: Characteristics of a good healthcare agent*

- ☐ Meets the state's legal requirements for a healthcare agent, including being over the age of 18.
- ☐ Will likely be available until your loved one's death (i.e., not someone who is close to death or has a terminal illness).
- ☐ Has a close, amicable relationship with your loved one; someone your loved one trusts with their life.
- ☐ Willing to take on the role of healthcare agent.
- ☐ Understands the significance of the healthcare agent role.
- ☐ Willing to discuss sensitive issues with your loved one.
- ☐ Shares your loved one's views and values regarding life, death, and medical treatments.
- ☐ Willing to follow all the stipulations in the living will, even if the agent does not agree with the stipulations.
- ☐ Willing to stand firm in the face of adversity if others do not agree with your loved one's wishes.

- ☐ Lives in close proximity to your loved one and is available to attend doctor's appointments or could travel to be close by if needed.
- ☐ Flexible and able to stay calm under pressure.
- ☐ Level-headed and mature.
- ☐ Not afraid to ask questions of healthcare providers.
- ☐ Not easily intimidated or overwhelmed by medical jargon or information. If available, it may be wise to choose someone who has a background in medicine or a basic understanding of medicine and healthcare. For example, if your loved one has 5 children who are otherwise equal, the individual with the medical background (e.g., nurse, physician, etc.) might be a natural choice to be the healthcare agent.
- ☐ Not someone your loved one picks out of guilt or obligation.
- ☐ Not someone who is your loved one's healthcare provider, a relative of a healthcare provider, an employee at a business or government agency that finances your loved one's healthcare, or anyone else who may have a conflict of interest. A person has a conflict of interest if competing interests might cause them to act against the welfare of your loved one.
- ☐ Common choices include a spouse, life partner, adult child, sibling, or trusted friend.

If you are close to the individual with Alzheimer's disease, you may be called upon to be their healthcare agent. If you are asked to take on this role, what responsibilities will you have? See the following checklist for some common responsibilities of a healthcare agent.

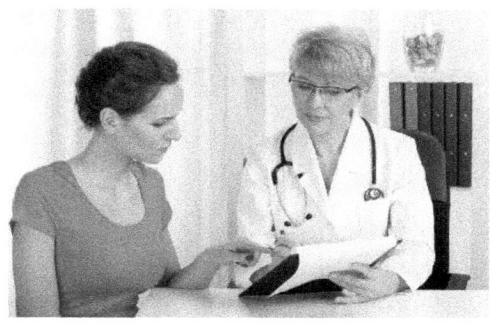

Credit: Photographee.eu

## *Checklist: Responsibilities of a healthcare agent*

### Before making healthcare decisions

- ☐ Discuss healthcare preferences with your loved one, including wishes for life-sustaining treatments. This should include preferences listed in your loved one's living will.
- ☐ Understand your loved one's current medications, including dosing and scheduling, as well as any allergies.
- ☐ Make sure physicians and other healthcare personnel as well as close family members or other trusted individuals have the most recent copies of all healthcare-related legal documents, such as the power of attorney, living will, and advance directives.

- ☐ Carry a copy of the durable power of attorney for healthcare with you to show to facilities in case they have misplaced the copy you gave them or they never received a copy.
- ☐ Ensure that the power of attorney document will be accepted by clinics, hospitals, and healthcare providers.
- ☐ Make sure the medical staff understands that you are the healthcare agent.

**Making decisions**

- ☐ Receive and understand information about your loved one's medical condition, including prognosis with and without treatment. Stay informed as your loved one's medical condition changes.
- ☐ Be present for support and consultation during medical tests and procedures. This includes attending regular doctor appointments as often as possible.
- ☐ Seek advice from medical professionals related to how you can be present for telehealth consults. Can you be included in the conference or appointment? Do you have to be with your loved one in person on a shared device? Or could you be at home on your own device?
- ☐ Access your loved one's medical records; because of HIPAA laws, the healthcare agent must present the durable power of attorney for healthcare document in order to be granted access to medical records.
- ☐ Discuss healthcare options with the medical team; understand the pros and cons of different

- treatment options. Write down information as needed.
- Be present for goals of care conversations. This is especially important toward the end of life when your loved one's symptoms start to become more severe.
- Write down questions to ask the physician, and ask them at the next opportunity. Prioritize more important questions first.
- Seek second opinions as needed.
- Get support from medical staff for decisions, including physicians, nurses, social workers, chaplains, members of the ethics committee, and others.
- Make healthcare decisions for your loved one; decisions should be similar to choices your loved one would make and in your loved one's best interest.
- After decisions have been made, pass the decisions on to healthcare workers and caregivers.
- Sign consent forms for medical procedures.

## Types of decisions

- Choose your loved one's physicians and other healthcare providers.
- Choose care facilities for your loved one.
- Approve a transfer of care between facilities or between physicians.
- Approve medical treatments that your loved one will receive, including but not limited to medications, therapy, and surgery.

- ☐ Withhold or withdraw medical treatments according to the living will or your loved one's religious or cultural views, such as withholding clinically administered nutrition and hydration or blood transfusions.
- ☐ Authorize or refuse participation in medical research; may also authorize that experimental treatments be stopped.
- ☐ Approve or revoke DNR or DNI (Do Not Intubate) orders after discussing the pros and cons with a physician.
- ☐ Choose whether your loved one will die at home or in a healthcare facility.
- ☐ Decide when to start or stop providing only comfort care, palliative care, or hospice care. Comfort care is care that helps your loved one feel more comfortable. This may include treatment for pain relief or other symptoms, taking a shower, or any other simple actions that help your loved one decrease their distress level. Palliative care is comfort care with or without treatments to help cure a disease. Hospice care is comfort care that is not focused on curative treatments. Hospice care is usually reserved for when the physician has indicated the individual has less than 6 months left to live. In all circumstances, your loved one should receive comfort care of some type. Do not allow your loved one's symptoms to go untreated just because they cannot communicate their level of distress.
- ☐ Decide when to start or stop providing only palliative care, comfort care, or hospice care.

- ☐ Give consent for organ donation and autopsy; your loved one's preference for this may be in the living will.

**Monitoring care**

- ☐ Know all of the medications your loved one takes, including doses and schedules. Keep track of all prescription and over-the-counter medications as well as vitamins and supplements. Make sure your loved one takes medications as prescribed.

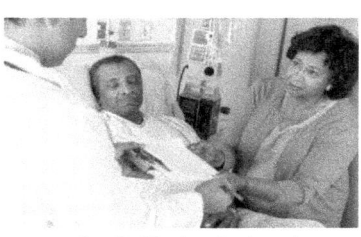
Credit: Monkey Business Images

- ☐ Make sure all prescribed treatments, tests, and procedures are being performed as ordered by the physician.
- ☐ Know what treatments should be started or stopped when your loved one is transferred to a new location or facility.
- ☐ Make sure pain and other symptoms are well managed.
- ☐ Provide comfort care as needed and allowed, such as giving ice chips, walking, assisting to the bathroom, etc.
- ☐ Be an advocate for your loved one if healthcare providers are not being responsive to requests.
- ☐ Monitor your loved one for signs of elder abuse, especially if your loved one is living in a long-term care facility. Signs of abuse or neglect include lack of control of symptoms or pain; worsening bed

sores; bruises, broken bones, or other indications of physical abuse; constant sedation above what is medically necessary; inadequate nutrition or hydration (other than at end of life); or fear of a particular person. For more information on signs of elder abuse, see *Home Safety Checklist Guide and Caregiver Resources for Medication Safety, Driving, and Wandering*.

- ☐ Post out-of-hospital DNR forms in your loved one's home, if desired.
- ☐ Know what to do or who to contact in case of a medical emergency.

**Other**

- ☐ Fill out applications or paperwork for long-term care facilities, hospital admission, doctor's appointments, etc.
- ☐ Inform the family about your loved one's condition.
- ☐ Understand who to contact if a mediator is needed to help resolve conflict between family members, especially conflict related to medical decisions.
- ☐ Do whatever is needed to stay in touch with your emotions, including talking to a counselor or clergy member.

# Advance Directives

Advance directives are legal healthcare documents that stipulate the actions your loved one wants physicians and other medical personnel to take during the course of their treatment. Some advance directives, such as the living will, can cover many situations and many healthcare actions. Other advance directives, such as the Do Not Resuscitate order, cover only one medical action in one specific circumstance. Usually no legal representative is named in an advance directive, but a healthcare agent or other healthcare representative should know and understand the contents of the advance directives put in place by your loved one. For more information about advance directives, see the Resources at the end of the book.

**Living Will**

The living will is a document that provides instructions about your loved one's desires for life-prolonging medical actions during specific circumstances. For example, if your loved one is declining rapidly and has no quality of life, the living will may stipulate that your loved one does not want to be subjected to artificial nutrition and hydration in order to prolong life. The following checklists provide basic information about living wills.

## *Checklist: Basics about a living will*

- ☐ Provides instructions for healthcare personnel about life-sustaining and other medical treatments.
- ☐ May also be called a directive to physicians, healthcare declaration, or medical directive.
- ☐ Can be completed without a lawyer in many states, although many states have specific rules about forms for advance directives.
- ☐ Most states have a witnessing requirement for the living will and other advance directives. Most states require two witnesses and/or a notary. Generally, the person's healthcare agent, family members, and healthcare providers cannot be witnesses.
- ☐ Becomes valid as soon as it is signed and does not have an expiration date.

- Only becomes effective once your loved one is no longer mentally competent and once they are near the end of life. Different states may have different requirements for this effective date.
- Outlines when specific medical treatments should be administered, withdrawn, or withheld. Although ethically they are similar, withholding medical treatment (or never starting it) tends to be an easier decision for healthcare agents than withdrawing medical treatment (or stopping it once it is started).
- Gives reassurance to the healthcare agent that they are following their loved one's wishes.
- Can be used to direct medical decisions if the healthcare agent is unavailable.
- Is very important for individuals who do not have anyone to be their healthcare agent.
- Cannot be used by a healthcare agent or family member to request medical records.
- Can be changed as many times as desired until your loved one is no longer legally competent.
- Does not constrain the actions of emergency medical personnel who are called to a home or long-term care facility. Emergency personnel are only responsible for keeping the individual alive until they are transferred to a medical facility.
- Having a living will in combination with a durable power of attorney for healthcare provides the greatest certainty

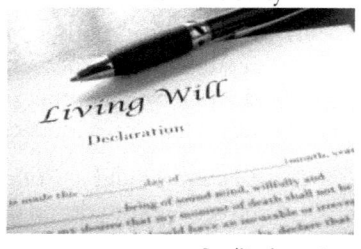

Credit: zimmytws

that your loved one's wishes for their medical care will be followed.

- [ ] If your loved one does not have a living will or other advance directives and is incapacitated, the healthcare agent, healthcare proxy, or guardian will need to make healthcare decisions without any input from your loved one.
- [ ] Keep in mind that a living will can provide guidance on your loved one's wishes for medical treatment, but it is also a legally binding document for medical personnel. Legally, they are required to follow the living will even if the healthcare agent feels that their loved one would make a different decision based on the circumstances. If your loved one has a trusted healthcare agent who will be available to make medical decisions, some individuals may choose to not have a living will. This should be discussed with your loved one, the healthcare agent, your loved one's physician, and your loved one's attorney.
- [ ] If your loved one chooses not to create a living will, your loved one should discuss and document their preferences for healthcare decisions with their healthcare agent and close family members.

## *Checklist: Medical treatments that may be covered in a living will*

- [ ] Do Not Resuscitate (DNR) order
- [ ] Do Not Intubate (DNI) order
- [ ] Use of clinically administered nutrition and hydration
- [ ] Organ, tissue, and body donation
- [ ] Use of dialysis

- ☐ Use of a ventilator or other artificial breathing method
- ☐ Use of a pacemaker or implantable cardioverter-defibrillator
- ☐ Use of aggressive treatments
- ☐ Options for a mental facility
- ☐ Palliative care
- ☐ Transfer to hospital
- ☐ Autopsy

## *Checklist: Responsibilities of the principal*

- ☐ Use the correct living will form as required by the state. An elder law attorney may be a good resource for this information. If your loved one spends significant time in more than one state, a living will should be completed for each state.
- ☐ Get information from a physician about the types of life-sustaining treatments that are available.
- ☐ Determine your loved one's preferences for advance directives such as Do Not Resuscitate forms, clinically administered nutrition and hydration, organ donation, and other medical treatments.
- ☐ Write the living will in such a way that it does not restrict the healthcare agent in unintended ways (e.g., outlining specific situations in which your loved one would not like to be placed on a ventilator).
- ☐ Create and sign the living will with the help of an attorney and witnesses.
- ☐ Store the living will in a safe but easily accessible location (NOT a safe deposit box), and tell the

- ☐ healthcare agent or other family members where the document is stored.
- ☐ Give regular healthcare providers, hospitals, the healthcare agent, family members, and other involved parties a copy of the living will.
- ☐ Discuss medical preferences listed in the living will with medical personnel, caregivers, the healthcare agent, and family members.
- ☐ Make sure chosen physicians will honor the instructions in the living will; if the physician refuses to honor some of your loved one's wishes, find a different physician who will.

## *Checklist: Situations to consider when deciding about life-prolonging medical procedures*

**Would my loved one want life-prolonging care if they:**

- ☐ Could no longer interact with friends and loved ones?
- ☐ Could no longer think or talk clearly?
- ☐ Could no longer respond to demands or requests?
- ☐ Could no longer walk independently?
- ☐ Could no longer contribute to their family's well-being?
- ☐ Could no longer control bowel and bladder activity?
- ☐ Could no longer independently perform activities of daily living (e.g., eating, toileting, dressing, etc.)?
- ☐ Had advanced dementia and could no longer recognize loved ones?
- ☐ Had significant brain damage?

- ☐ Were confined to the house or bed?
- ☐ Were in constant discomfort (pain, nausea, etc.) that could not be controlled with medication?
- ☐ Were in a permanent coma?
- ☐ Were a severe emotional or financial burden on their family?
- ☐ Required dialysis to stay alive?
- ☐ Required clinically administered nutrition and hydration to survive?
- ☐ Required mechanical ventilation to survive?
- ☐ Required frequent defibrillation to survive?

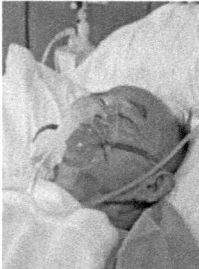
Credit: kessudap

If your loved one has stipulated circumstances in which they felt that life would no longer be worth living, they may provide instructions for when they want their healthcare agent to sign a Do Not Resuscitate (DNR) or Do Not Intubate (DNI) order. Instructions for when to sign a DNR order are one of the most common items included in a living will.

## Do Not Resuscitate and Do Not Intubate

Unless your loved one has a DNR order, medical personnel are legally and ethically required to perform heroic efforts to bring your loved one back to life if they undergo cardiac or respiratory arrest. In the absence of a DNR order, not using heroic efforts in these circumstances could instigate a court hearing and potential removal of their medical license. With a DNR order, medical personnel can be liable for legal action if they do perform heroic efforts to bring the individual back to life, although most courts will not prosecute medical staff, especially emergency personnel, for performing cardiopulmonary resuscitation (CPR) if they were unaware of the DNR order. Your loved one's wishes for a DNR or DNI order may be stated in the living will, but the actual DNR and DNI orders require a separate legal document. The following checklist provides details about DNR and DNI orders.

## *Checklist: Basics about DNR and DNI orders*

- ☐ If your loved one has a DNR order, physicians and other medical personnel will not use heroic efforts to bring your loved one back to life if they undergo cardiac arrest (the heart stops beating) or respiratory arrest (your loved one stops breathing). This primarily refers to administration of CPR but may also refer to mechanical ventilation (using a machine to breathe for your loved one) and the use of a defibrillator (a machine that produces an electric shock to start the heart beating again).

- ☐ A DNR order is not an order not to treat the patient. It simply withholds CPR. Other treatments, such as pain medication, antibiotics, comfort care measures, and even aggressive treatment of a disease can all still be given when a DNR order is in effect.

- ☐ A DNR order may also be called an Allow Natural Death (AND) form in some states.

- ☐ If your loved one has a DNI order, physicians and other medical personnel will not intubate your loved one. Intubation involves putting a tube down the throat to aid in breathing or to hook up mechanical ventilation/artificial breathing.

- ☐ A DNR or DNI order can be requested by your loved one or your loved one's healthcare agent, but the order must be signed by a physician.

- A DNR or DNI order can be signed or revoked at any time.
- Medical personnel must have access to a signed DNR or DNI order in your loved one's medical records for it to be honored.
- If your loved one is in the hospital, the DNR or DNI order should be prominently displayed by your loved one's bed. If it is not, make sure the medical staff have a copy of the DNR or DNI order and ask them to post a copy in your loved one's room.
- A DNR order is only effective in a hospital or doctor's office. If your loved one is seriously ill and wants a DNR order at home where emergency medical personnel may provide care, they will need an out-of-hospital DNR order posted in their home; this may be on an official form, wallet card, or bracelet.
- If an out-of-hospital DNR order is not obviously posted, emergency medical personnel and bystanders will not be held legally responsible if they perform CPR on your loved one.

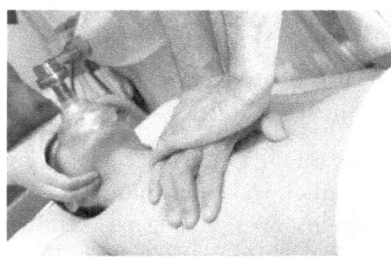

Credit: sfam_photo

Signing a DNR order is a significant step and should not be taken lightly. The following checklists offer some common reasons to sign, not sign, or revoke a DNR order. Remember that each individual's circumstances are different, so you may not want to sign a DNR for your loved one under all of these circumstances. In addition, there may be other circumstances not listed that may provide sufficient reason to sign (or not sign) a DNR order.

## *Checklist: When should my loved one have a DNR order?*

- ☐ If they are likely a few days or hours away from death.
- ☐ If they are frail and CPR may cause more damage (e.g., broken ribs) than good.
- ☐ If they are in a permanent coma with little or no chance of recovery.
- ☐ If they have little chance of leaving the hospital even if successfully revived.
- ☐ If successful CPR has little chance of helping them recover for more than a few days.
- ☐ If they have a low quality of life, such as very late-stage Alzheimer's disease, and medical treatments are unlikely to restore quality of life.
- ☐ If they are bed-bound and have lost the ability to swallow (e.g., they cannot consume food or drink through the mouth).
- ☐ If they are in substantial pain due to a terminal condition that is not relieved by pain medication.
- ☐ If they are on mechanical ventilation with no chance of recovery.
- ☐ If they are in multi-organ failure (kidney, liver, heart, etc.).
- ☐ If a physician states that they would recommend a DNR order.
- ☐ Under any circumstances stated in the living will. Your loved one should consider circumstances

under which they would or would not want a DNR order signed, including circumstances listed in these checklists, and record their wishes in their living will.

## *Checklist: When should my loved one NOT have a DNR order?*

- ☐ If they are going into surgery. (Active DNR orders are often suspended for the duration of the surgery.)
- ☐ If they recover from a life-threatening illness or disease.
- ☐ If they are months or years away from death.
- ☐ If they have a good chance of recovery after treatment.
- ☐ If successful CPR will allow the individual to leave the hospital and regain some quality of life.

The choice of whether to approve a DNR order is a major decision that will be one of the hardest the healthcare agent has to make. However, if your loved one has reached a stage of disease in which they are close to death and have no chance of recovery, a DNR order may save them from a prolonged, painful dying process. If your loved one has given stipulations for the use of a DNR or DNI order in their living will, those orders should be followed explicitly. Although it is hard to lose a loved one, sometimes the best thing you can do for them is let them die naturally if they are already near death.

### Clinically Administered Nutrition and Hydration

Clinically administered nutrition and hydration is primarily used when your loved one is no longer able to swallow enough food and water to maintain adequate nutritional intake. Individuals with Alzheimer's disease often lose the ability to swallow properly, and swallowing often leads to aspiration, or the intake of food or liquid into the lungs. This can lead to infections, particularly pneumonia, which can be fatal in frail, elderly individuals. In fact, aspiration pneumonia is the leading cause of death for individuals with Alzheimer's disease. For individuals who are unable to swallow properly, clinically administered nutrition and hydration may be required to sustain life and prevent infection. To learn more about clinically administered nutrition and hydration, see the following checklist.

## *Checklist: Basics about clinically administered nutrition and hydration*

- ☐ Clinically administered nutrition and hydration can be categorized into parenteral nutrition and enteral nutrition.

- ☐ Parenteral nutrition is nutrition that is administered directly into the veins via an intravenous (IV) tube.

- ☐ Parenteral nutrition is often used to administer hydration (water) and electrolytes (sodium, calcium, chloride, magnesium, potassium, phosphorus, etc.).

- ☐ Enteral nutrition is nutrition administered directly into the stomach via a small tube inserted through the nose (short-term) or through an incision in the abdominal cavity (long-term). This is typically called a "feeding tube."

- ☐ Enteral nutrition is used to administer calories via a liquid formula that contains fats, proteins, and carbohydrates. The

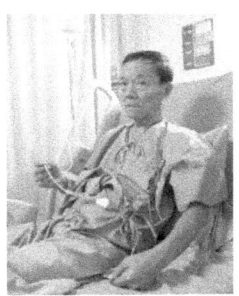

Credit: stockphoto mania

caloric content and nutritional makeup of the formula is chosen based on the individual's needs.

- [ ] Your loved one's living will can state when nutrition should be administered, when it should be withheld, and when it should be withdrawn.
- [ ] Common reasons to administer clinically administered nutrition and hydration include temporarily controlling what enters the stomach (such as after surgery or to help heal stomach ulcers) or providing a source of nutrition for individuals who cannot swallow (such as some Alzheimer's patients and quadriplegics).
- [ ] Clinically administered nutrition and hydration are often withheld or withdrawn if the individual is close to death and the nutrition will not help them recover or give them a better quality of life.
- [ ] Experts agree that for individuals who are close to death, withholding nutrition and hydration does not cause pain or feelings of hunger or thirst.
- [ ] Experts agree that for frail individuals near the end of life, providing nutrition and hydration may cause more harm than good because it puts stress on the failing kidneys and digestive system.
- [ ] Individuals who are close to death who do not receive clinically administered nutrition and hydration may live as long as two weeks or more before death, but they may also pass away within a day or two, depending on their physical state.

## Organ, Tissue, and Body Donation

Some individuals would like their healthy organs or tissues donated to others who need them, and some individuals choose to have their entire body donated for medical research or medical teaching. If your loved one would like to donate their organs, tissues, or body, the following checklist provides some important information to consider. For more information about organ donation, see websites listed in the Resources at the back of the book.

## *Checklist: Basics about organ, tissue, and body donation*

- ☐ The living will can state whether your loved one wants their healthy organs and/or tissues donated to others who may benefit from them. This can also be stated on your driver's license in many states.

- ☐ Commonly donated organs include the heart, intestines, kidneys, liver, lungs, and pancreas.

- ☐ Commonly donated tissues include blood vessels; bone, ligament, nerve, and skin tissue; cartilage and connective tissues; and the eyes/corneas.

- ☐ In order to donate organs, the organs must receive blood until they can be harvested. Therefore, your loved one may need to be put on mechanical ventilation until the harvesting procedure is complete, even if they had a DNI order. The living will should state that your loved one understands the need for this temporary intervention.

- ☐ The living will can also state if your loved one wants their body donated for research or to a medical teaching facility for students.

- ☐ If your loved one wants to donate their body, their will must state where they want their body donated and they need to make arrangements with the facility before their death. In addition, many institutions require a fee for accepting a donated body due to lack of funding.

- ☐ Donation of organs, tissues, or body usually means that an autopsy would not be beneficial for your loved one, although individuals with Alzheimer's disease may specifically have only their brain autopsied to identify characteristic lesions associated with Alzheimer's disease.

- ☐ Some individuals who are old or terminally ill may not have organs that are suitable for donation.
- ☐ Even if their organs are harvested, your loved one's body can still be shown at the funeral.

**Other Directives**

Many other medical directives can be given in a living will, and a living will can be changed to reflect your loved one's diagnosis of Alzheimer's disease, provided your loved one makes the changes while they are still legally competent. The following checklist provides descriptions of a few less-common medical directives.

*Checklist: Basics about less-common medical directives*

- ☐ **Dialysis.** Dialysis is used to remove toxins from the blood when the kidneys no longer work properly. Dialysis is usually performed at least three times per week for individuals with minimal kidney function, and it often takes 3-4 hours for each session, leaving the individual exhausted. Individuals on frequent dialysis usually have a fistula or shunt to ease access to the blood vessels for dialysis. If not cared for properly, these access points can become infected. However, many individuals are on dialysis for years with minimal complications. Without dialysis, individuals with failing kidneys die quickly from too many toxins in the blood. For individuals who are dependent on dialysis, stopping dialysis usually results in death within 1-2 weeks.

- **Ventilation.** Ventilation is used to help a person breathe when they are not able to breathe adequately on their own. Ventilation can be invasive or noninvasive. Invasive ventilation includes intubation, or placing a tube down the throat to deliver oxygen directly to the lungs. This requires the person to be sedated. Noninvasive ventilation does not use intubation. Instead, oxygen is delivered through the mouth and nose with the use of a mask and positive air pressure. Sedation is not required for noninvasive ventilation. Ventilation could also include other types of machines such as CPAP or BiPAP machines, which are typically used for sleep apnea and other similar disorders. These machines are typically noninvasive. Note that a DNI order does not prevent the medical team from using noninvasive ventilation.
- **Pacemaker or implantable cardioverter-defibrillator.** Some individuals have a pacemaker or implantable cardioverter-defibrillator due to chronic heart problems or an abnormal heart rhythm. Individuals who have these may choose to have them turned off when they are at or near the end of life. This may or may not be done in conjunction with signing the DNR order.
- **Medical treatments.** Some individuals with progressive Alzheimer's disease may choose not to receive aggressive treatments such as radiation or chemotherapy after a cancer diagnosis, or even not to receive antibiotics after being diagnosed with an infection. These treatments may cause your loved one's physical or mental state to worsen, or they could prolong life when the quality of life is already low.

- **Care facilities**. Individuals with Alzheimer's disease slowly lose their mental capabilities, often leaving them depressed, violent, or suicidal. Some individuals with Alzheimer's disease stipulate in their living will when they would be willing to be admitted to a mental or long-term care facility, including a memory care facility, and which facility they would choose to be admitted to.

- **Palliative care.** Many individuals with Alzheimer's disease may opt to receive only palliative care in the advanced stages of the disease. *Palliative care* refers to care that relieves suffering and provides comfort measures such as pain medication or medication to relieve constipation. Palliative care or comfort care should be provided at all times, regardless of whether your loved one has decided to allow or forego more aggressive treatments. Palliative care helps your loved one maintain their dignity and quality of life until their natural death. Palliative care is often given at home through hospice care, although palliative care can and should be started long before your loved one enters hospice care. For more information about palliative and hospice care, see the Resources at the end of the book.

- **Transfer to hospital.** If given a choice, most individuals state that they would rather die at home than in a hospital. Therefore, some individuals state in their living will that they do not want to be transferred to a hospital when they are near death, or they state the circumstances under which they would choose to go to a hospital. For individuals with Alzheimer's disease, transferring locations may cause confusion and hasten death, so in the late stages of the disease they should not be moved to a new location, even if it is their own home, unless it is medically necessary.

☐ **Autopsy.** The only way to definitively diagnose Alzheimer's disease is to do a brain autopsy after death to identify characteristic brain lesions associated with Alzheimer's disease. Some individuals may state in their living will or in their last will and testament whether they would like to have an autopsy performed after their death. Note that the cost of an autopsy is often charged to the patient if it is elective.

# Physician Orders for Life-Sustaining Treatment (POLST)

Many of the advance directives summarized in this chapter can be stated in a simple form called a Physician Orders for Life-Sustaining Treatment, or POLST (also called MOLST, or Medical Orders for Life-Sustaining Treatment). The POLST form is usually filled out in the presence of the physician or other qualified medical personnel as well as your loved one or your loved one's legal representative. The POLST form is then posted by your loved one's bed, usually on a brightly colored piece of paper (usually pink), so that all medical personnel involved in your loved one's care are aware of the form and your loved one's choices for treatment.

The POLST form contains instructions from your loved one or your loved one's legal representative regarding end-of-life care, including use of CPR, clinically administered nutrition and hydration, and other medical interventions. The POLST form can also indicate the presence of an advance directive or living will document. Instructions given on the POLST form are regarded as direct physician orders and must be followed by all medical personnel. For more information about POLST, see the Resources at the end of the book.

# Chapter 4:
# Legal Documents for Finances

In addition to being unable to make healthcare decisions, your loved one with Alzheimer's disease will likely be unable to make good financial decisions as they progress through the disease. This is because they are unable to understand basic financial concepts, recognize poor financial decisions and scams, and remember to pay bills. Therefore, choosing someone who can handle their financial affairs both during their lifetime and after their death will be vital to their financial stability.

## Durable Power of Attorney for Finances

A durable power of attorney for finances is created to name a single individual or group of individuals who will be allowed to make financial decisions for your loved one. Although likely not as important as choosing a good healthcare agent, choosing a qualified individual to make financial decisions is important for making sure your loved one's financial needs are taken care of while they are still alive. See the following checklists for important information about the durable power of attorney for finances.

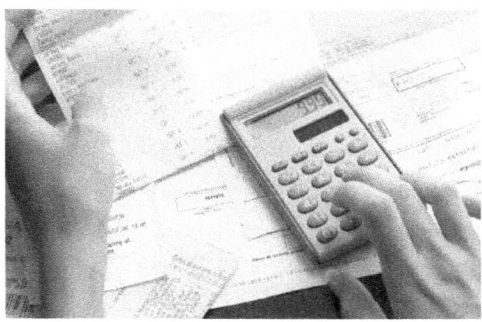

Credit: bikeriderlondon

## *Checklist: Basics about a durable power of attorney for finances*

- ☐ The individual creating the durable power of attorney for finances is called the principal. In this book, your loved one with Alzheimer's disease is assumed to be the principal.
- ☐ The individual named to make financial decisions for the principal is called the attorney-in-fact.
- ☐ The attorney-in-fact is only allowed to make financial decisions, not healthcare decisions, for your loved one.
- ☐ The durable power of attorney for finances is valid as soon as it is signed, but the attorney-in-fact usually does not have any responsibilities before your loved one becomes legal incompetent except for specific duties stated in the document.
- ☐ The durable power of attorney for finances is valid for both individual transactions (e.g., selling a specific piece of property as designated in the document) and for global management of finances (e.g., after the principal is incapacitated).
- ☐ The durable power of attorney for finances can be revoked or changed at any time, as long as your loved one is still legally competent.
- ☐ The durable power of attorney for finances document will not allow the attorney-in-fact to obtain your loved one's medical records.
- ☐ If your loved one does not have an attorney-in-fact and becomes incapacitated, you or another individual will need to petition the court for conservatorship.

## *Checklist: Responsibilities of the principal*

- ☐ Determine whether any state laws restrict the choice of attorney-in-fact.
- ☐ Choose an attorney-in-fact based on desired characteristics of an attorney-in-fact. Make sure the chosen agent is willing to accept this responsibility. Usually having only one active attorney-in-fact at a time is best to prevent disagreements about property.
- ☐ Choose an alternative attorney-in-fact if the original attorney-in-fact is unavailable or is unwilling to serve.
- ☐ Stipulate any restrictions on the attorney-in-fact, such as when they can make decisions (e.g., after the principal is legally incompetent) or which specific transactions they are responsible for.
- ☐ Create and sign the durable power of attorney for finances document.
- ☐ Distribute copies of the durable power of attorney for finances to banks, investment companies, insurance companies, utility companies, and other companies that the attorney-in-fact will interact with financially.
- ☐ Keep a copy of the durable power of attorney for finances document in an easily accessible place at home, and tell the attorney-in-fact and close family members or other trusted individuals where to find the document.
- ☐ Discuss financial responsibilities, obligations, and wishes with the attorney-in-fact.
- ☐ Discuss living trusts and the last will and testament with the attorney-in-fact, even if they are not the executor of the will or trustee.

- ☐ Tell family members who the chosen attorney-in-fact is and why.
- ☐ If one attorney-in-fact becomes unwilling or unable to serve, or if your loved one wishes to revoke the agent's power, your loved one will need to create a new document and destroy all old documents.

## *Checklist: Characteristics of a good attorney-in-fact*

- ☐ Meets the state's legal requirements for attorney-in-fact, including being over the age of 18.
- ☐ Has a close and amicable relationship with your loved one.
- ☐ Is willing to take on the role of attorney-in-fact.
- ☐ Lives in close proximity to your loved one.
- ☐ Is knowledgeable about financial matters and keeps good financial records.
- ☐ Is financially responsible, which will ensure that your loved one's bills are paid on time.
- ☐ Has similar personal financial views as the principal. For example, if the principal is generally opposed to taking on debt, they probably wouldn't want to choose an attorney-in-fact who has tens or hundreds of thousands of dollars in debt.
- ☐ Understands your loved one's goals and wishes for their finances and is willing to follow those goals and wishes.
- ☐ Understands your loved one's financial portfolio and knows where important financial documents are kept.
- ☐ Is trusted by close family members.
- ☐ If your loved one is married, they will likely choose their spouse as their attorney-in-fact.

- ☐ Other common options for attorney-in-fact are an adult child, sibling, trusted friend, family lawyer, or bank.
- ☐ Although it is possible to name more than one individual as the attorney-in-fact, usually it is best to name only one person to avoid conflicts between them when making financial decisions.
- ☐ If the family is likely to have arguments over financial decisions and assets, using a neutral third party as the attorney-in-fact is often the best choice.

## *Checklist: Responsibilities of an attorney-in-fact*

- ☐ Manage finances while your loved one is still living; after death, financial decisions and distribution of property fall to the executor of the will.
- ☐ Read the directions given in the durable power of attorney document and follow what it says.
- ☐ Make sure all relevant parties (banks, utility companies, investment brokers, insurance companies, etc.) have a copy of the durable power of attorney for finances.
- ☐ Ensure that the power of attorney document will be accepted by banks, utility companies, and other financial institutions.
- ☐ Make decisions that are in the best interest of your loved one, not the attorney-in-fact or your loved one's family members.
- ☐ Discuss financial goals and priorities with your loved one.
- ☐ Make sure that your loved one's financial needs are being met.
- ☐ Find out if your loved one is eligible for financial services, including pensions, disability, Social

Security, Medicare, Medicaid, Veterans benefits, housing assistance, or food stamps (SNAP); help your loved one apply for these services and benefits. For a benefits checkup website, see the Resources at the end of the book.

- ☐ Fill out government reports required for government benefits such as Social Security income, Veteran's benefits, and disability income.
- ☐ Get legal advice about Medicaid eligibility from an elder law attorney.
- ☐ Involve your loved one in financial decisions for as long as possible.
- ☐ Research your loved one's past financial decisions to determine how they would have acted under different circumstances.
- ☐ Use common sense when making financial decisions for your loved one.
- ☐ Oversee bank accounts and balance checkbooks; make sure bank accounts are receiving interest and have no or low fees.
- ☐ Keep accurate and honest financial records.
- ☐ Pay bills, taxes, and other expenses on time.
- ☐ Purchase or sell property based on your loved one's previous purchasing and selling habits or their financial needs.
- ☐ Collect rent or unpaid debt.
- ☐ Keep real estate in good condition.
- ☐ Make investments carefully.
- ☐ Purchase insurance policies as needed, and cancel unnecessary insurance policies.

- ☐ Keep your loved one's property safe through the use of a safe deposit box, insurance, a security system, locks, and other safety measures.
- ☐ Keep personal financial holdings separate from your loved one's financial holdings.
- ☐ Avoid conflicts of interest (i.e., situations in which a decision may benefit another party but harm your loved one).
- ☐ Resist borrowing or spending money for personal reasons or loaning money to others from your loved one's estate. Note that it is very easy for an attorney-in-fact to drain your loved one's financial resources because they have complete control of your loved one's accounts. Steps should be taken to prevent this, such as requiring the attorney-in-fact to maintain detailed records of how money is being spent. This record may be useful if you have to seek legal action against the attorney-in-fact.
- ☐ Give money away only if it is within your loved one's normal pattern of giving (e.g., birthday gifts for grandchildren, annual donations to a charity, etc.).
- ☐ Do not charge a fee for financial management services, unless the power of attorney document permits it.
- ☐ Be aware of and work to prevent financial abuse or scams that your loved one may be subject to.

## Last Will and Testament

In contrast to a durable power of attorney for finances that names someone to manage property before your loved one's death, the last will and testament states how property should be distributed after your loved one's death. While not every single possession needs to be listed individually in the will, large items or items with great sentimental value should be specifically designated for distribution. The checklists below provide some basics about the last will and testament as well as common items listed in the will and how they are frequently distributed. Remember that this list is not be inclusive, and distribution ideas are examples only.

## *Checklist: Basics about a last will and testament*

- ☐ The last will and testament, or will, provides instructions for how an individual wants their estate distributed after their death.
- ☐ The person writing the will is called the testator. After death, they are referred to as the decedent. In this book, your loved one with Alzheimer's disease is assumed to be the testator.
- ☐ The individual named to distribute property as listed in the will is called the executor of the will. The executor is usually a spouse, adult child, or family lawyer, but may be a close friend or other trusted individual.
- ☐ Individuals who will receive property listed in the will are called beneficiaries. Beneficiaries are usually your loved one's spouse, children, grandchildren, siblings, friends, and favorite charities.
- ☐ Your loved one must be legally competent to write a valid will, and they must be over the age of 18.
- ☐ For the courts to recognize a will as valid, it must be written (as opposed to verbal) and contain at least two witness signatures.
- ☐ The will is only valid after your loved one's death.
- ☐ The will can be revoked or changed at any time, as long as your loved one is still legally competent.

- An amendment to the will can also be written; this is called a codicil.

- Your loved one's significant assets should be listed in the will (see *Checklist: Items commonly listed in the will*) unless beneficiaries are stated directly on the account (such as a savings account or insurance policy).

- Your loved one may be able to make a simple will (limited property and few beneficiaries) online or with purchased computer software, but complicated wills (a large estate with many beneficiaries) should be created with the help of a lawyer.

- For property to be distributed, the will must be filed with the probate court, which is the legal system that handles property distribution after someone's death.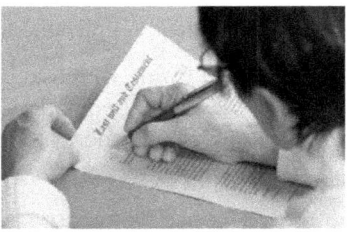

  Credit: NotarYES

  Most wills will not ever appear in court; if written well, the executor will be allowed to distribute your loved one's property out of court.

- If the will is not written or witnessed properly, if someone contests the will, or if your loved one does not have a will, the will may go through a lengthy probate process. In these cases, probate court can be expensive and time consuming.

- Any documents that go through probate court, such as a will, become public record. Therefore, anyone can read the contents of the will and beneficiaries. To avoid probate court, a living trust can be created.

- Even if a living trust exists, everyone should have a will to distribute property not listed in the trust, including guardianship of minor children and distribution of personal items such as clothing and furniture.
- If your loved one dies without a will, the court will appoint an administrator of the estate to handle the distribution of property.

## *Checklist: Responsibilities of the testator*

- Choose an executor of the will based on the desired characteristics of an executor. Make sure the executor is willing to accept this responsibility.
- Choose an alternative executor if the original executor is unavailable or is unwilling to serve.
- Determine which items should be listed in the will and name beneficiaries for each item. Use specific names of beneficiaries rather than broad categories such as "nieces and nephews."
- Choose alternate beneficiaries if the original beneficiary cannot accept the assets. Alternate beneficiaries should include an "ultimate beneficiary," the beneficiary (or beneficiaries) that will receive the estate if all the original and alternate beneficiaries are deceased or not available. The ultimate beneficiary is typically not a person. It could be a charitable organization, business or university, or other organization that is likely to still be in place after the testator's death.
- Create and sign the last will and testament. State clearly in the document that this is a will.
- Distribute copies of the last will and testament to interested parties, including the executor, key family members, and a family lawyer.

- ☐ Keep a copy of the last will and testament in an easily accessible place at home and tell the executor and close family members where to find the document.
- ☐ Discuss distribution of property with the executor.
- ☐ If the primary executor becomes unwilling or unable to serve, or if your loved one wishes to change executors or change stipulations in the will, your loved one will need to create a new document and destroy all old documents.
- ☐ Review the will whenever there is a major change in your loved one's circumstances, such as a birth, death, marriage, or divorce in the family (see also Checklist: Reasons to review legal documents).

## *Checklist: Items commonly listed in the will*

- ☐ **Guardianship for minor children.** One of the most important statements in a will is who will be the guardian of any minor children still in the household. Each child should have an individual or couple named as a guardian, even if the same individual or couple is named for every child. Common choices for guardianship of minor children include a surviving parent, grandparent,

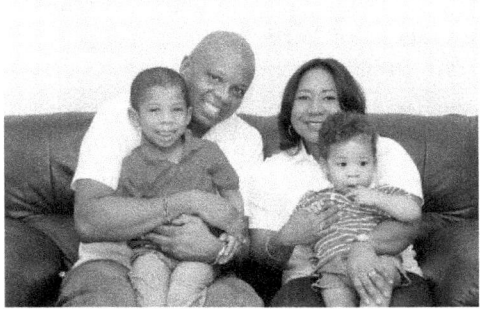

Credit: Maria Maarbes

aunt or uncle, godparent, or trusted friend. Be sure to discuss this choice with the chosen guardian.

- [ ] **Guardianship for adult children with disabilities.** Similar to minor children, the will needs to state who will become guardian of an adult child with a disability. Similar options for guardianship are available as for minor children. However, because of the disability, some individuals may decline guardianship, so confirm that the individual is willing to become guardian before adding their name to the will.

- [ ] **Pets.** Although not as vital as naming a guardian for children, the will should also contain instructions for who should care for any pets that remain after your loved one's death. For most individuals, this will be a cat or dog, but it may also include animals such as horses, cattle, sheep, goats, snakes, mice, gerbils, birds, and other less common pets or farm animals.

- [ ] **Real estate, such as a primary residence, vacation home, or rental property.** If your loved one is married, real estate, especially a primary residence, is often passed to the surviving spouse. If no surviving spouse remains, real estate frequently goes to the oldest child or is sold and the proceeds split evenly among children. If your loved one does not have children, real estate may go to other family members or friends.

- [ ] **Vehicles.** Vehicles such as cars, trucks, boats, RVs, ATVs, and others may be left to the surviving spouse, a child or grandchild who needs transportation (e.g., a grandchild going to college), or an individual who shares a similar hobby (e.g., a boat could be given to a friend who shares a love of fishing); donated to a local charity; or sold and the proceeds divided among heirs.

- **Cash.** Cash is one of the most versatile possessions to pass on. First, available cash should be used to pay any debts or outstanding bills. Once debts are paid, cash can be distributed to family, friends, charities, or other organizations. Note that individuals who are listed as beneficiaries or joint owners of cash accounts such as checking or savings accounts usually have priority over any distribution listed in the will.

- **Investments.** Investments such as stocks, bonds, and mutual funds are often passed down to the surviving spouse, children, grandchildren, or siblings. They can also be gifted to some charities. Some investments allow you to list a beneficiary. If a beneficiary is listed on the investment, the investment does not need to be listed in the will.

- **Insurance payouts.** Insurance policies such as life insurance have a payout upon the policy holder's death. Most insurance policies that pay benefits on death will require you to list a beneficiary on the policy itself. However, if a beneficiary is not listed, the policy benefits can be distributed through the will. Common beneficiaries include a surviving spouse, children, or grandchildren.

- **Jewelry.** Jewelry, especially expensive or heirloom jewelry, should be included in the will to prevent family arguments. Wedding rings are often willed to the oldest daughter or granddaughter. A father's watch may go to the oldest son. Some family members may state a preference for receiving a specific piece of jewelry. Jewelry can also be sold and the proceeds distributed to the heirs or donated to a charity.

- **Furniture.** If furniture is expensive or handmade, specific individuals in the family may want to take possession of those items. Basic furniture could be given to grandchildren who are just starting their own homes or donated to a local charity for families in need.

- **Household items.** Unless someone needs or wants a specific household item, common household items are often donated to a local charity or sold in an estate sale.

- **Clothing.** Most clothing items are donated to a local charity or given to someone who requests specific clothing items. A wedding dress may be passed down to a daughter or granddaughter.

- **Tools.** Tools may be passed on to children or grandchildren who need them. Unwanted tools may be donated to a local charity or sold in an estate sale.

- **Ownership in a business.** If your loved one owns a family business, the will can name the individual(s) who will take over your loved one's ownership shares and responsibilities. The transfer of responsibility will likely take place before your loved one's death. However, ownership shares in the business may be passed on before or after

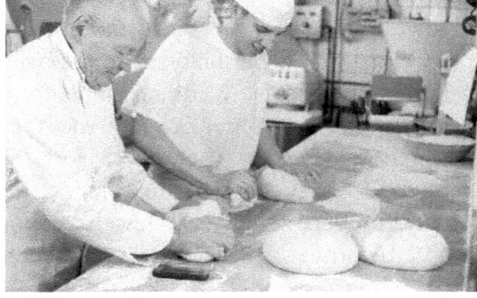

Credit: racord

death. Ownership shares are often transferred to the individual who took over the business or split among surviving children.

- **Trusts.** If desired, a will can be used to set up a testamentary trust for managing your loved one's money after their death. This is common if the beneficiaries are still minors (under 18 years old) at the time of your loved one's death.

- **Funeral and burial arrangements.** If your loved one has purchased a burial plot or has specific instructions about the use of a particular funeral home, church, order of service, or headstone engraving, these should be included in the will and discussed with family members.

- **Other.** Other items of monetary or sentimental significance should be included in the will as well. These items can be willed to a specific individual or charity or sold at an estate sale.

Individuals who have a last will and testament should also name an executor of their will in the will document as well as a successor executor in case the original executor becomes incapacitated. Characteristics of a good executor and responsibilities of an executor are listed below.

## *Checklist: Characteristics of a good executor of the will*

- Meets the state's legal requirements for executor, including being over the age of 18 and having no prior felony convictions.
- A trusted individual, such as a spouse, adult child, family lawyer, close friend, or bank.
- Is willing to be executor of the will.
- Has the time and skills needed to properly execute the will.

- ☐ Is organized and meticulous when dealing with important documents.

## *Checklist: Responsibilities of an executor of the will*

- ☐ Oversee the distribution of your loved one's property according to the will. The executor of the will has no legal authority while your loved one is still alive.
- ☐ Contact beneficiaries to attend a reading of the will.
- ☐ Consult an attorney about the probate process.
- ☐ File legal documents in probate court to receive an official executor document that allows them to distribute the estate.
- ☐ Attend court appearances related to your loved one's will, if needed.
- ☐ Advocate with the court to have your loved one's assets distributed according to the will.
- ☐ Settle debts owed by your loved one and collect on debts owed to your loved one.
- ☐ Appraise the value of your loved one's assets.
- ☐ File paperwork related to transferring property from your loved one to beneficiaries.
- ☐ Oversee the sale of real estate or other assets as listed in the will.
- ☐ Oversee an estate sale or donation of items to charity.
- ☐ File estate and other taxes for the decedent as necessary.

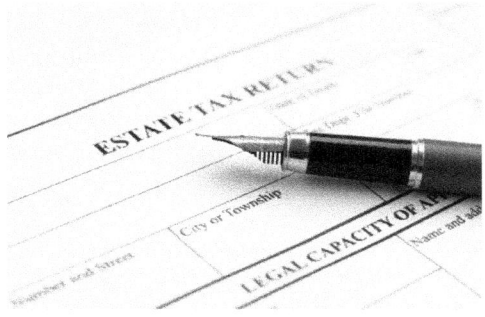
Credit: alexscopje

# Trusts

In addition to a last will and testament, property can be transferred to beneficiaries through a trust. Trusts can seem very complicated at first, but they can help shelter your loved one's assets and protect certain assets from taxes if executed correctly. Before forming a trust, talk to a financial planner, lawyer, or trust department at your local bank to help you decide which type of trust will be best for your loved one. The checklists below include several facts about trusts.

## *Checklist: Terms related to trusts*

- ☐ **Trust.** A document that creates an agreement between a grantor, trustee, and beneficiaries for how the grantor's property will be distributed to beneficiaries either during the grantor's lifetime or after the grantor's death.

- ☐ **Grantor.** The grantor is the person who creates the trust. The grantor may also be called the trustor, settler, or donor. In this book, your loved one with Alzheimer's disease is assumed to be the grantor.

- ☐ **Trustee.** The trustee is the person who manages the trust. The grantor is often named the trustee. The trustee can also be a spouse, adult child, family lawyer, or friend. Often a neutral third party such as a trust department at a bank will be named trustee. Successor trustees should also be named in case the primary trustee is unable to complete their duties. (See *Checklist: Characteristics of a good trustee*.)

- ☐ **Decedent.** The grantor after their death.
- ☐ **Beneficiary.** The individuals or other parties that receive property through the trust. Beneficiaries are usually the grantor's spouse, children, grandchildren, or friends. Beneficiaries can also be charitable organizations.
- ☐ **Property.** The items that are placed in the trust. The property in the trust may also be called the principal. (See *Checklist: What to put in a trust*)
- ☐ **Surviving spouse.** The spouse of the grantor that is still alive after the grantor's death.

## *Checklist: Types of trusts*

- ☐ **Living Trust.** A living trust is a trust created and managed during your loved one's lifetime. Your loved one usually retains control of a living trust (i.e., they are the trustee) during their lifetime as long as they are mentally competent. Property in a living trust can be transferred to beneficiaries both while your loved one is still alive and after your loved one's death, depending on the stipulations in the trust. Because a living trust is a legal document describing how property in the trust is to be distributed, it does not have to go through probate court. This is the most common type of trust and the most advantageous for individuals with Alzheimer's disease.
- ☐ **Testamentary Trust**. A testamentary trust is a trust that is created upon execution of your loved one's will. Therefore, a testamentary trust must be

described in your loved one's last will and testament. Because a testamentary trust is part of the will, it is created when the will goes through probate court after your loved one's death. This makes a testamentary trust more public than a living trust.

- **Revocable Trust.** A revocable trust is a trust that can be modified or dissolved during your loved one's lifetime. For example, real estate named in the trust can be sold and new real estate purchased for the trust, or money in an account named in the trust can be added to or spent. In addition, beneficiaries can be changed in a revocable trust. The designation of revocable trust generally only refers to a living trust (i.e., a revocable living trust) because testamentary trusts are always revocable until your loved one's death.

- **Irrevocable Trust.** An irrevocable trust is a trust that cannot be modified once it is created. Therefore, when your loved one transfers property to an irrevocable trust, they no longer have ownership rights to that property. Living trusts can be irrevocable (i.e., an irrevocable living trust), and both living and testamentary trusts become irrevocable upon your loved one's death.

- **Purpose-based trusts.** Trusts can be created for a specific purpose, such as managing property or money for a minor child until they reach the age of 18, managing property or money for an adult child with a disability, protecting assets from Medicaid or lawsuits, protecting assets for children from a previous marriage, avoiding certain types of taxes such as an estate tax or gift tax, exempting life insurance payouts from estate taxes, and giving to charitable organizations. Because the types of purpose-based trusts and the tax laws they affect are so diverse, you should speak to a qualified trust agent, lawyer, or financial planner to discuss which trust is right for your loved one.

## *Checklist: What to put in a trust*

- ☐ **Real estate.** Primary residences, vacation homes, rental properties, undeveloped land, corporate buildings, or any other real estate owned by your loved one can be placed in a trust.

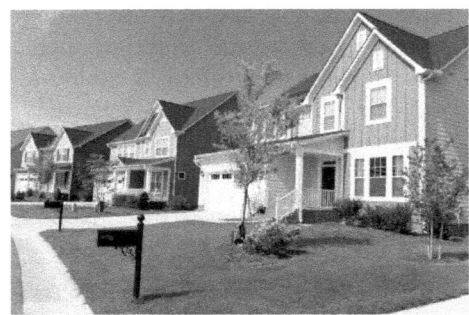

Credit: Konstantin L

- ☐ **Cash.** Cash accounts such as checking accounts, savings accounts, and certificates of deposit can all be placed in a trust.

- ☐ **Investments.** Investments such as stocks, bonds, and mutual funds can be placed in a trust.

- ☐ **Insurance.** Insurance policy payouts can name a trust as the beneficiary. Most commonly, life insurance policies are placed in an irrevocable living trust. Depending on the stipulations in the trust and the type of life insurance policy, this may exempt the policy payout from estate taxes, leaving the beneficiaries with the entire payout rather than only a portion of the payout.

- ☐ **Valuable property.** Other valuable property such as vehicles, jewelry, and other items with monetary or sentimental value can be placed under the ownership of the trust.

- ☐ Remember that only property placed in the trust can be managed by the trust. (See *Checklist: How do I help my loved one create a trust?*)

## *Checklist: How do I know if my loved one needs a trust?*

- ☐ If your loved one has a small estate and no minor or disabled children, a will is often sufficient for distribution of assets.
- ☐ If your loved one plans to leave their entire estate to their surviving spouse, a will is sufficient for distribution of assets.
- ☐ If your loved one wants to avoid the costs and time required for probate court, create a trust. Although trusts may be more expensive to create up front, they are less expensive to execute after your loved one's death. The opposite is true for wills. Depending on the length and complexity of the probate process, a will could end up costing significantly more than a trust overall.
- ☐ If your loved one does not want the contents of their estate to be made public, create a trust.
- ☐ Even if your loved one's estate is small, they have no minor or disabled children, and they have a simple estate distribution plan, a trust is often better than a will because it avoids the probate process. However, the cost vs. benefit of a will vs. a trust will differ based on the size of the estate and state laws. A trusted attorney or financial planner can help you determine what would work best for your loved one's situation.

- ☐ If your loved one has a large estate, especially an estate that is larger than the current amount that is exempt from estate taxes ($13.61 million in 2024), they should create a trust.
- ☐ If your loved one wants to shelter their estate from Medicaid asset requirements, they will need to form an irrevocable living trust at least 5 years before they apply for Medicaid assistance.

## *Checklist: How do I help my loved one create a trust?*

- ☐ Like other legal documents, your loved one must be mentally competent to create a trust. Therefore, you should start this process immediately after the diagnosis of Alzheimer's disease if you have not already done so.
- ☐ Identify someone who can help your loved one create a trust document. This may be a lawyer, financial planner, or trust department at a bank.
- ☐ Identify the items your loved one would like to place in the trust. Gather legal paperwork such as deeds, titles, and other proof of ownership.
- ☐ Once the trust is created, manually change the owner of every account, property, and any other item that your loved one wants in the trust to the name of the trust (e.g., instead of the account owner being Joe Smith, the owner should be changed to the Joe Smith Living Trust).
- ☐ Any property that is not manually transferred to the name of the trust will not be included in the trust.
- ☐ Any property not in the trust should have the beneficiary updated to the name of the trust. The trust will then designate how that property is distributed upon the grantor's death.

- ☐ Designate beneficiaries for every item in the trust or otherwise provide instructions for how the property in the trust should be distributed.
- ☐ For revocable trusts, update the document as often as needed. For example, your loved one may need to update the trust document if a new grandchild is born.
- ☐ Also remember that even if your loved one has a trust, they still need to have a last will and testament for all their possessions that are not named in the trust, such as clothing and household items. Also, guardians of minor children or adult children with disabilities will need to be named in a will rather than a trust.

Once a trust is created, a trustee will be responsible for managing the trust. Choosing a good trustee is vital to having the trust managed honestly and according to your loved one's wishes. The checklists below describe characteristics of a good trustee and responsibilities of a trustee.

## *Checklist: Characteristics of a good trustee*

- ☐ Meets the state's legal requirements for trustee, including being over the age of 18; however, your loved one will want to choose someone young enough to oversee the trust for many years if needed.
- ☐ A trusted individual, such as the grantor or a spouse, adult child, family lawyer, close friend, bank, or trust company. If you choose a family member, choose wisely so as not to drive a wedge between the trustee and other family members. More than one trustee can be appointed if needed (such as all the adult children of a couple), although

doing so is not recommended because it may cause conflicts that cannot be resolved.

- ☐ Is willing to be trustee.
- ☐ Has time to manage the trust.
- ☐ Understands the contents of the trust and how property should be managed.
- ☐ Understands investing, accounting, and legal responsibilities.
- ☐ Understands money management principles.
- ☐ Has integrity, accountability, and good judgment.
- ☐ Is responsible, organized, and mature.
- ☐ Is financially secure (to minimize risk of the trustee misusing trust funds for their own purposes).
- ☐ If choosing a bank or trust company, choose one that has a good reputation, longevity, sufficient capital, and liability insurance.

## *Checklist: Responsibilities of a trustee*

- ☐ Carefully manage the property in the trust based on your loved one's wishes.
- ☐ Seek the good of your loved one rather than the good of the beneficiaries.
- ☐ Weigh the importance of different options to determine which option is closest to your loved one's wishes; be unbiased when making decisions about the trust.
- ☐ Oversee management of investments, property, and other trust accounts.
- ☐ Make prudent investments with your loved one's money.

- ☐ Buy or sell property.
- ☐ Rent or lease property.
- ☐ Pay bills as needed from the trust cash accounts.
- ☐ File and pay income tax for the trust as needed.
- ☐ Keep records and perform accounting procedures for the trust accounts.
- ☐ Keep up with changing laws that affect the trust and the responsibilities of the trustee.
- ☐ Recognize problems and seek the advice of professionals as needed.
- ☐ Maintain effective communication with your loved one and beneficiaries of the trust.
- ☐ Disburse money and property to beneficiaries.
- ☐ Maintain confidentiality about sensitive trust information.

Also from Omega Press

# Save Money, Live Healthy

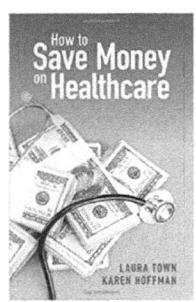

*How to Save Money on Healthcare* provides answers to the following questions and more:

- **What types of insurance are available to me?** Explore public and private insurance options, learn how they work, and find out who is eligible for them.
- **How can I use my personal savings to pay for care?** Learn about the types of personal wealth, the rules associated with them, and the way they are used to pay for healthcare.
- **What out-of-pocket alternatives exist?** Discover different options to help pay your out-of-pocket medical expenses without draining your savings.
- **How can I manage my medical bills?** Find out how to detect and correct billing errors and what your options are if you are unable to pay your medical bills.

# Chapter 5: Other Legal Documents

Although not as common, several other legal documents may be used to help your loved one make healthcare, financial, or other decisions. Some of these documents become either inactive or active based on your loved one's mental competence or death, some are appointed by a physician, and some are appointed by the court system if your loved one has neglected to make legal documents before their incapacitation.

## Power of Attorney

In addition to the durable power of attorney, the two other kinds of power of attorney are the general power of attorney and the springing power of attorney.

### General Power of Attorney

The *general power of attorney* (usually just called a power of attorney) is someone who has been appointed to make financial decisions for another person. Often, a power of attorney is set up for a specific purpose, which is stated in the power of attorney document; once that purpose is fulfilled, the document is no longer valid. For example, if you live in one state but hold property in another state, you may set up a power of attorney authorizing someone in the other state to sell your property for you.

A distinguishing factor of a general power of attorney compared to a durable power of attorney is that it is only viable while the grantor is legally competent. Once the grantor has been declared incompetent, the general power of attorney document is no longer viable. Therefore, a power of attorney that is not durable is not recommended for individuals with Alzheimer's disease.

### Springing Power of Attorney

In contrast to a power of attorney, a *springing power of attorney* is only effective once the individual is no longer mentally competent. While this may seem like a good option for someone with Alzheimer's disease, the process of declaring someone legally incompetent can be difficult because different people may have different ideas about what constitutes competence versus incompetence. During the time it takes to declare your loved one officially incompetent, your loved one is required to continue making their own financial and healthcare decisions when they shouldn't be. Therefore, using a durable power of attorney is best for individuals with Alzheimer's disease.

## Healthcare Proxy

In some states, a healthcare agent is also called a healthcare proxy or medical power of attorney. However, a healthcare proxy or healthcare surrogate can also refer to someone who is appointed by a physician to make medical decisions for an individual who is medically incapacitated but doesn't have a healthcare agent or a court-appointed guardian. In this regard, the individual has no control over whom the physician chooses to be their healthcare proxy. The physician often chooses a close loved one who is with the individual, such as a spouse or adult child. Once appointed, the healthcare proxy has similar responsibilities to the healthcare agent. To avoid needing a healthcare proxy, your loved one should sign a durable power of attorney for healthcare while they are still mentally competent.

## Conservatorship/Guardianship

Another alternative for individuals who do not have a durable power of attorney for healthcare or finances is to have the court appoint a conservator or guardian to make healthcare and financial decisions. In some states, the terms conservator and guardian mean the same thing. However, traditionally a conservator is a court-appointed individual who oversees an incapacitated individual's financial matters, and a guardian is a court-appointed individual who oversees an incapacitated individual's personal matters, such as healthcare decisions and where to live. The courts will state the powers granted to the conservator or guardian. Usually, the court will only appoint a conservator or guardian if testing finds that the individual is legally incompetent.

If your loved one became incompetent before realizing they needed power of attorney documents or simply refused to sign a power of attorney for healthcare or finances, you or your loved one's family members can petition the court for rights of conservatorship or guardianship. The court will first have to determine whether your loved one is mentally incompetent, and then the court will appoint someone to be the conservator or guardian. This may or may not be the person who petitioned the court for conservatorship or guardianship. Once this ruling is in place, the appointed person then has the same rights and responsibilities as a durable power of attorney for healthcare and/or a durable power of attorney for finances, depending on the court's ruling. If your loved one doesn't agree with the ruling, they have the right to object to the conservatorship or guardianship. In addition, if there appears to be conflict among family members for the choice of guardian or conservator, the court may choose a neutral party rather than a family member.

Although appointing a conservator or guardian is helpful, it should only be used as a last resort if your loved one is incapacitated and does not have durable power of attorney documents in place, because the court proceedings can take as long as one year to complete. In addition, if a conservator or guardian is appointed before a durable power of attorney can be located or identified, the conservator or guardian has legal authority, not the person named in the durable power of attorney.

## Guardianship of Minor Children

In addition to appointing someone to be guardian for your loved one, the courts may need to appoint a guardian for your loved one's minor children or adult children with disabilities if your loved one becomes unable to care for them. A last will and testament is used to dictate guardianship of minor children after your loved one's death, and a clause can be added that the same individual should care for the children if your loved one becomes incapacitated.

In addition, other legal documents can be used specifically for the purpose of transferring guardianship while your loved one is alive but incapacitated. For this purpose, your loved one will need to create a nomination of guardianship (also called a parental appointment of a guardian) or joint guardianship document. A nomination of guardianship document names the person (or people) that your loved one chooses to have guardianship of their children if your loved one becomes incapacitated. A joint guardianship document allows your loved one to transfer legal rights to another individual while your loved one is still alive and to also keep parental rights until your loved one's death; this is the recommended legal document for individuals with Alzheimer's disease.

Accepting guardianship of minor children or an adult with a disability is a major responsibility. Therefore, choosing an appropriate guardian is of utmost importance. In general, to ease the transition for the child, appoint the same guardian in a guardianship document as is listed in the last will and testament. In addition, if guardianship will go to a couple, both the husband and wife should be listed in the guardianship document. An alternative guardian should also be listed in case the primary guardian is unavailable.

Once the guardian has begun their duties, they will need to care for that child as if the child is their own, including meeting the financial responsibilities that come with raising the child, unless the child's parent has made financial provisions for their care through a will or trust. The checklist below indicates things to consider when choosing a good guardian for children.

## *Checklist: Things to consider when choosing a good guardian for children*

- ☐ Does the individual meet the legal requirements of a guardian, including being over the age of 18?
- ☐ Is the individual willing to accept guardianship of all of your loved one's children? Or would the children be placed in different homes?
- ☐ Does your loved one's child prefer one particular individual to be their guardian if the parents become incapacitated?
- ☐ Does the individual have a genuine interest in the well-being and care of your loved one's children?
- ☐ Is the individual physically, emotionally, and financially able to care for the children?
- ☐ Is the individual willing to spend their own money to care for your loved one's children?
- ☐ Does the individual get along well with your loved one's children?
- ☐ Will the individual provide a stable home and family life for your loved one's children?
- ☐ Does the individual share the morals, values, and beliefs that your loved has tried to instill in their children?

- ☐ Will the individual discipline your loved one's children in the same manner your loved one would discipline them?
- ☐ Is the individual willing to accept full responsibility for the child's actions even if they get in trouble with the law?
- ☐ If living with this individual, would your loved one's children be able to attend the same school they did previously? Or would they have to change school systems?
- ☐ If the child (or adult) has a disability, does the individual have the time, energy, and skill needed to care for a person with a disability?

# Administrator

If your loved one dies without a last will and testament, the courts will appoint an administrator to oversee the distribution of your loved one's estate. The administrator may or may not be someone your loved one would have chosen. In most states, the court will name your loved one's spouse as the administrator. If your loved one has no spouse, the next of kin is usually selected. In general, the administrator has the same responsibilities as a named executor. However, an executor may have additional duties compared to an administrator based on the stipulations of the will (such as the sale of real estate). The administrator will also have to post bond for the estate, which is a cost determined by probate court. The bond is a fee to ensure that the administrator will follow state laws when executing the estate. This cost is often waived if your loved one has a will and a named executor.

# Government Benefits

An individual acting as the durable power of attorney

for finances does not have the legal right to manage income from Social Security or Veterans benefits. If your loved one is eligible to receive benefits from these sources, the government names the agent who will manage these benefits. A representative payee is named to manage Social Security benefits, and a VA fiduciary is named to manage Veterans benefits. The government may appoint the same individual or entity as the durable power of attorney for finances, but they may also choose someone else instead.

## Social Media Will

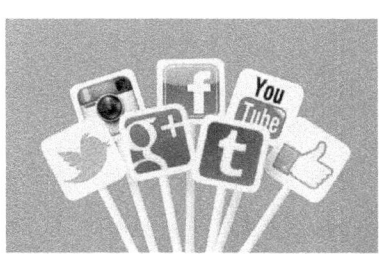

Credit: Bloomus/Shutterstock.com

As we move further into the digital age, more individuals are opening social media accounts on Facebook, Instagram, TikTok, and others. The privacy laws governing social media accounts keep anyone other than the original owner from accessing the account. If your loved one has any social media accounts, they should consider writing a social media will. First, your loved one should consult the privacy policies for each social media site. Then, in the will, write how the loved one would like the account handled after incapacitation or death based on the privacy policies of the site. Some sites may allow a page to remain open as a memorial, or the site may require that your loved one's page be closed or canceled. Your loved one should provide the executor of their social media will with a list of accounts, login IDs, and passwords. The executor should also obtain a copy of your loved one's death certificate because some companies require this for someone else to make changes to the account.

# Ethical Will

Although an ethical will is not technically a legal document, it can be used to pass on values, memories, and beliefs to those left behind just as much as a last will and testament can be used to pass on physical possessions. An ethical will is usually a letter or video that provides a last message to close family members and friends about the things that hold most value for your loved one. It can include statements of personal or religious beliefs, hopes and dreams for children or grandchildren, words of encouragement, lessons your loved one has learned in life, or forgiveness or apologies for past hurts. A loved one who is young with small children may want to write letters for children to open on important dates such as birthdays, graduations, weddings, etc. Ethical wills can also be used to try to mend broken relationships. For individuals with Alzheimer's disease who will slowly lose their mental capabilities, writing an ethical will is a great way to preserve memories and solidify relationships before your loved one is no longer able to communicate.

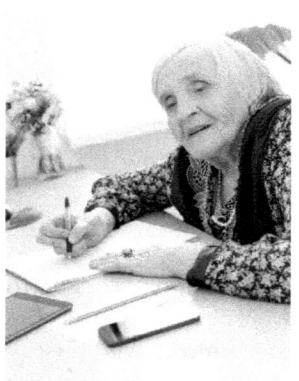

Credit: Yeko Photo Studio

# Chapter 6: Dealing with Conflict

Caring for a loved one with Alzheimer's disease brings with it may decisions, complications, and stresses. For many families, daily decisions about healthcare, finances, and other responsibilities are a heavy burden that often brings out the worst in everyone. These problems are magnified in blended or dysfunctional families. Dealing with family conflict adds more stress to an already stressful situation, especially for family members who are involved in caring for your loved one in a legal capacity. My friend Amy and I are both only children, so we did not have any disputes with family members. However, there are a million stories of families being torn apart because of decisions made by one sibling or parent that the other family members did not agree with. The checklists below note common causes of disagreements and provide ways to resolve or prevent conflicts.

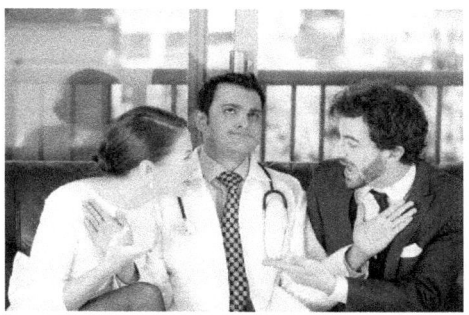

Credit: PathDoc

## *Checklist: Common causes of conflict*

- ☐ Family members have different opinions about the best choices for medical care, especially at the end of life. This is especially common between a spouse and adult children.

- ☐ Family members disagree about what they think your loved one would want in a particular situation, including both healthcare and financial decisions.
- ☐ Family members disagree about who should be the primary caregiver for your loved one, or one family member refuses to participate in caregiving.
- ☐ A family member is not carrying an equal burden of caring for your loved one or feels like they are carrying the whole burden of care.
- ☐ A family member is resented for living far away and not contributing to your loved one's care.
- ☐ Family members disagree on who should provide housing for your loved one if your loved one can no longer live alone.
- ☐ Family members disagree on who should be your loved one's physician or which long-term care facility they should move into.
- ☐ Children from blended families disagree on how your loved one should be cared for.
- ☐ Children from a first marriage resent involvement of a spouse or children from a second marriage.
- ☐ Family members allow childhood conflicts or rivalries to infiltrate the decision-making process concerning your loved one's care.
- ☐ Family members disagree about or don't fully understand your loved one's physical and mental limitations.
- ☐ Family members have different opinions about the distribution of assets, especially for expensive items or items with great sentimental value.
- ☐ A family member insists that they want their inheritance now before your loved one's death.

- ☐ A family member wants to "borrow" money from your loved one's estate.
- ☐ Family members disagree about how to pay for your loved one's care.
- ☐ Family members disagree about the contents of a legal document.
- ☐ Family members disagree about how to deal with scams your loved one has fallen prey to.
- ☐ Family members feel anger, fear, frustration, resentment, helplessness, or grief over your loved one's condition.
- ☐ A family member is in denial about your loved one's condition. Similarly, if your loved one is in denial about their condition or diagnosis, this can also lead to conflict.

## *Checklist: Strategies to prevent or resolve conflict*

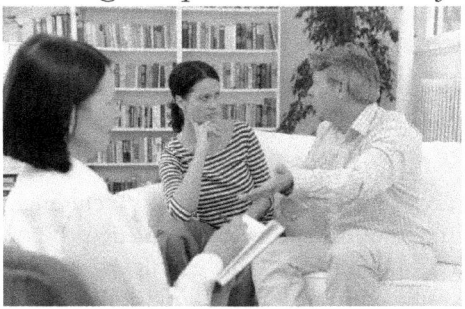

Credit: Konstantin L

- ☐ Listen carefully to family members' opinions, and respect their opinions. Keep an open mind and try to understand their point of view.
- ☐ Keep lines of communication open between family members. Try not to exclude family members from

this discussion, even if they live far away or are known for their poor choices and irresponsibility.

☐ Keep family members informed about your loved one's condition as it changes.

☐ Schedule regular face-to-face meetings for the family to discuss changes in your loved one's situation. Also use these meetings as a forum for anyone to voice feelings of experiencing caregiver burnout.

☐ Talk honestly about your feelings and burdens with other family members or friends. Sometimes sharing the burden can help lighten the load for everyone.

☐ If you are the legal representative, understand your legal rights when making decisions about your loved one's healthcare and/or finances while also allowing other family members to share their opinions and provide insight when making big decisions, such as when and where to move your loved one from their home.

☐ Express appreciation for the care that others are providing.

☐ Make a list of caregiving tasks, including how much time, money, and effort is needed to complete the task. Divide tasks as evenly as possible among family members based on skills and availability. Tasks may include cooking, cleaning, providing hygiene care, doing grocery shopping, performing home maintenance, paying bills, driving to appointments, and many others.

☐ Plan for anticipated changes in your loved one's needs as the disease progresses.

- ☐ Avoid physically or verbally attacking others who have a different opinion than you do.
- ☐ Try not to blame others for bad situations; don't criticize others for not participating in your loved one's care or not performing care "correctly."
- ☐ Resolve childhood conflicts between family members to allow everyone to participate in decisions and caregiving without letting past issues disrupt the current situation.
- ☐ Seek help from a neutral third party when disagreements occur. For healthcare disagreements, consult your loved one's physician or other medical professional. For financial disagreements, consult your loved one's attorney or trustee (if the trustee is not a family member). For other disagreements, consult a counselor, pastor, mediator, social worker, or shared friend. Websites that list mediators by state are provided in the Resources.
- ☐ Encourage family members to join a support group for families of individuals with Alzheimer's disease.
- ☐ Hire help to provide caregiving services or take care of household tasks.
- ☐ If you live far away, offer to help in any way you can. Offer to provide emotional support to caregivers through phone calls, letters, or cards. Offer financial support if needed. Visit as your schedule allows.
- ☐ Make sure all family members and caregivers are taking care of themselves by getting regular sleep, nutritious meals, and adequate exercise.

# Conclusion

The creation of legal documents is a detailed matter that should not be taken lightly. The selection of a healthcare agent, attorney-in-fact, executor, or trustee requires careful consideration, and the named representative will have heavy responsibility placed on them after committing to the job. In addition, determining healthcare choices for the end of life and determining how property will be distributed will require critical thinking and thorough planning. If your loved one has been diagnosed with Alzheimer's disease, many of these decisions will become too hard for them once the disease progresses. Therefore, creating legal documents as soon as possible after diagnosis is essential. Both you and your loved one will feel a weight lifted off your shoulders once major decisions about the future have been made and these legal documents are in place.

# About the Authors

## Laura Town

Laura Town has authored numerous publications of special interest to the aging population. She has expertise in the field of finance as a co-author on *Finance: Foundations of Financial Institutions and Management* published by John Wiley and Sons, and she has contributed to several online nursing courses and texts. She has

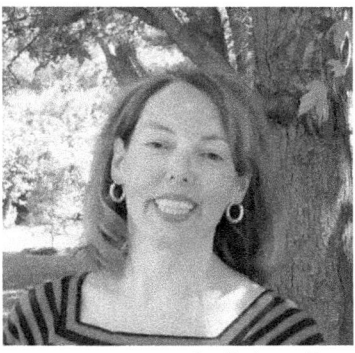

Credit: Laura Town

also written for the American Medical Writers Association, and her work has been published by the American Society of Journalists and Authors. As an editor, Laura has worked with Pearson Education, Prentice Hall, McGraw-Hill Higher Education, John Wiley and Sons, and the University of Pennsylvania to create both on-ground and online courses and texts. She is the past president of the Indiana chapter of the American Medical Writers Association. Laura's book *Dementia, Alzheimer's Disease Stages, Treatments, and Other Medical Considerations* is one of Book Authority's top ten best-selling print books about dementia and top 100 best audiobooks about dementia of all time.

# Karen Hoffman

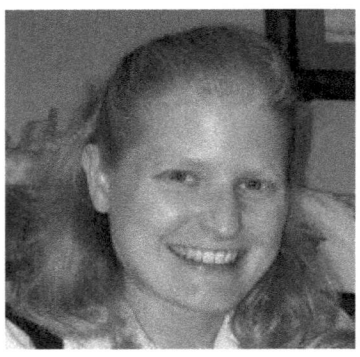

Credit: Karen Hoffman

Karen Hoffman received a Ph.D. in Pharmacology from the Department of Pharmacology and Experimental Neurosciences at the University of Nebraska Medical Center in Omaha, NE, where she was the recipient of an American Heart Association fellowship and several regional and national awards for her research on G protein-coupled receptor signaling in airways. She then pursued post-doctoral research projects at the University of North Carolina-Chapel Hill and the University of Kansas Medical Center, again receiving fellowships from the PhRMA Foundation and the American Heart Association, respectively. She has published research in the American Journal of Pathology, Journal of Biological Chemistry, and Journal of Pharmacology and Experimental Therapeutics. In 2012, Karen joined the editorial staff at WilliamsTown Communications, an editing firm that specializes in educational products for undergraduate- and graduate-level students. At WTC, Karen specializes in producing educational products related to the sciences and healthcare. In addition, Karen is board-certified for editing life sciences (BELS-certified).

# A Note from the Authors

Thank you for purchasing our book! Worldwide, nearly 55 million people suffer from Alzheimer's disease or other forms of dementia, and that number is expected to increase significantly within the next 15 years. In the United States, approximately 6.7 million people have Alzheimer's disease, and that is expected to increase to 13 million by the year 2050.

Despite these large numbers, you may feel alone. I (Laura) know that when I started caring for my father, who had early-onset Alzheimer's disease, I felt alone. Although my father has passed away, I am haunted by what he suffered and how difficult it was to care for him. However, now I know that there are people, resources, and organizations that can help others going through this same struggle.

We recognize that caregivers have emotional, physical, and financial challenges. We hope that the information in the Alzheimer's Roadmap series will ease some of your stress. The legal documents discussed in this book will help you prepare for that inevitable day when your loved one is no longer able to make their own decisions about healthcare and finances. In addition, we have included resources at the end of each book to provide additional information to help you through this process.

If you have any questions, please reach out to Laura via LinkedIn: https://www.linkedin.com/in/lauratown/. We would appreciate it if you would take the time to review our book on Amazon, as our book's visibility on Amazon depends on reviews.

# Additional Titles from Laura Town and Karen Hoffman

Alzheimer's Roadmap series:

*Long-Term Care Insurance, Power of Attorney, Wealth Management, and Other First Steps*

*Dementia, Alzheimer's Disease Stages, Treatment Options, and Other Medical Considerations*

*Coping with Dementia*

*Enhancing Activities of Daily Living*

*Home Safety Checklist Guide and Caregiver Resources for Medication Safety, Driving, and Wandering*

*Paying for Healthcare and Other Financial Considerations*

*Home Care, Long-term Care, Memory Care Units, and Other Living Arrangements*

*Caregiver Resources: From Independence to a Memory Care Unit*

*Nutrition for Brain Health: Fighting Dementia*

*Final Steps: End of Life Care for Dementia*

Other titles:

*How to Save Money on Healthcare*

*Where Should Mom Live?*

*Caring for Aging Parents: Navigating the Journey*

# Resources

**Information about Alzheimer's Disease**

Alzheimer's Association
225 N. Michigan Avenue, Fl. 17
Chicago, IL 60601
Phone: 800-272-3900
Website: http://www.alz.org

Alzheimer's and Related Dementias Education and Referral Center (ADEAR)
Phone: 800-438-4380
Email: adear@nia.nih.gov
Website: https://www.nia.nih.gov/health/alzheimers-and-dementia/about-adear-center

Alzheimer's Foundation of America
322 Eighth Avenue, 16th Fl.
New York, NY 10001
Phone: 866-232-8484
Email: info@alzfdn.org
Website: www.alzfdn.org

**Information about Legal Advice or Lawyers**

Administration on Aging Eldercare Locator
Phone: 800-677-1116
Email: eldercarelocator@n4a.org
Website: https://eldercare.acl.gov/Public/Index.aspx
*Find connections for legal assistance and many other topics

American Bar Association
321 North Clark Street
Chicago, IL 60654
Phone: 800-285-2221

Email: Service@americanbar.org
Website: https://www.americanbar.org/
*Provides legal information related to many topics

National Academy of Elder Law Attorneys
Email: naela@naela.org
Website: https://www.naela.org/
*Lists all certified elder law attorneys in the U.S.

National Institute on Aging
Building 31, Room 5C27
31 Center Drive, MSC 2292
Bethesda, MD 20892
Phone: 800-222-2225
Email: niaic@nia.nih.gov
Website: http://www.nia.nih.gov/
Specific helpful websites:
https://www.nia.nih.gov/health/topics/legal-and-financial-issues-alzheimers
*Provides a list of resources for legal and financial issues

National Center on Law & Elder Rights
Website: https://ncler.acl.gov/
*Provides information about legal issues and legal resources

Justice in Aging
1444 Eye Street, NW Suite 1100
Washington, DC 20005
Phone: 202-289-6976
Website: https://justiceinaging.org/
*Provides limited free legal information

## Information about Organ Donation and Other Advance Directives

Donate Life America
701 East Byrd Street, 16th Fl.
Richmond, VA 23219
Phone: 804-377-3580
Website: www.donatelife.net

Health Resources and Services Administration
Phone: 888-275-4772
Email: donation@hrsa.gov
Website: www.organdonor.gov

National POLST (Physician Orders for Life-Sustaining Treatment)
208 I Street NE
Washington, DC 2002
Phone: 202-780-8352
Email: info@polst.org
Website: https://polst.org/form-patients/

Put It In Writing
American Hospital Association
155 North Wacker Drive
Chicago, IL 60606
Phone: 800-424-4301
Website: https://www.aha.org/system/files/2018-01/putitinwriting.pdf

The Living Bank
4545 Post Oak Place, Suite 340
Houston, TX 77027
Phone: 800-528-2971
Website: www.livingbank.org

## Information about Resolving Family Conflict

Alzheimer's Association
Website: https://www.alz.org/help-support/community/support-groups
*Search for local support groups

Elder Decisions
30 Walpole Street
Norwood, MA 02062
Phone: 617-621-7009
Email: info@elderdecisions.com
Website: www.elderdecisions.com
*Mediators will travel to your location

Mediate.com
Website: https://www.mediate.com/index.cfm
*Provides links for finding mediators by state/city and country

Mediation.org
1292 High Street #1015
Eugene, OR 97401
Website: https://www.aaamediation.org/
*Search for mediators by state/city/zip code

## Other

AARP
601 E Street, NW
Washington, DC 20049
Phone: 888-OUR-AARP (888-687-2277)
Website: http://www.aarp.org/
*Information for individuals over age 50

National Council on Aging Benefits CheckUp
251 18th Street South, Suite 500
Arlington, VA 22202
Website: https://www.benefitscheckup.org/
*Helps find government benefits that you qualify for

National Hospice and Palliative Care Organization
1731 King Street
Alexandria, VA 22314
Phone: 703-837-1500
Website: https://www.nhpco.org/patients-and-caregivers/
*Provides information about hospice services

# Reference List

Alzheimer's Association. (2021). Retrieved from https://www.alz.org/

American Bar Association. (2021). Retrieved from https://www.americanbar.org/

American Health Lawyers Association. (2008). A guide to legal issues in life-limiting conditions. Retrieved from https://www.hindshospice.org/uploads/1/5/2/5/15252368/legalguidetolifelimitingillness.pdf

Bryant, K. (n.d.). 37 types of trusts used to protect assets from creditors, the government, and other predators. Retrieved from http://www.eldercarelawjacksonville.com/2012/04/25/types-of-trusts-protect-assets/

Burroughs, A. (2011). When your client has Alzheimer's. Retrieved from http://wealthmanagement.com/financial-planning/when-your-client-has-alzheimer-s

California POLST forms. (2021). Retrieved from https://capolst.org/polst-for-healthcare-providers/forms/

Candito, J. (2011). Executor or administrator? What's the difference? Retrieved from http://blueashattorney.com/2011/10/executor-or-administrator-whats-the-difference/

CaregiverStress.com. (2021). Retrieved from https://www.caregiverstress.com/

Caring.com. (2021). How to deal with caregiving-related family conflicts. Retrieved from https://www.caring.com/caregivers/family-caregivers/#how-to-deal-with-caregiving-related-family-conflicts

Casey, J. (2008). How to hire an elder law attorney. Retrieved January 2020 from http://alzheimers.about.com/lw/Health-Medicine/Geriatric-Health/How-to-Hire-an-Eldercare-Attorney.htm

Celebrations of Life. (n.d.). Ethical wills/Legacy letters. Retrieved from http://celebrationsoflife.net/ethicalwills/

Consumer Financial Protection Bureau. (2013). Managing someone else's money: Help for agents under a power of attorney. Retrieved from https://files.consumerfinance.gov/f/201310_cfpb_lay_fiduciary_guides_agents.pdf

Dimick, C. (2011). Sorting out advance directives. *Journal of AHIMA*, 82(1): 26–30.

Family Caregiver Alliance. (2020). Caregiving and sibling relationships: Challenges and opportunities. Retrieved from https://www.caregiver.org/caregiving-and-sibling-relationships-challenges-and-opportunities

FindLaw. (2021) How to establish guardianship of a child FAQs. Retrieved from https://www.findlaw.com/family/guardianship/how-to-establish-guardianship-of-a-child-faqs.html

Fisher Center for Alzheimer's Research Foundation. (2021). Retrieved from http://www.alzinfo.org/

The Florida Bar. (2021). Consumer pamphlet: Do you have a will? Retrieved from https://www.floridabar.org/public/consumer/pamphlet011/

The Free Dictionary. (2021) Executors and administrators. Retrieved from https://legal-dictionary.thefreedictionary.com/Executors+and+Administrators

Guest, C (2012). The trustee...picking a trustee...Part 1. VA Estate Planner. Retrieved from https://vaestateplanner.wordpress.com/2012/03/19/the-trusteepicking-a-trusteepart-1/

Higuera, V. (2017). Complications of Alzheimer's disease. Retrieved from https://www.healthline.com/health/alzheimers-disease-complications#Overview1

Just Health and Family Law. (2010). Guardianship agreements. Retrieved January 2020 from http://www.justhealthandfamily.com/guardianship-agreements.html

Life Issues Institute. (n.d.). Planning for future medical decisions: How to prepare a personalized living will. Retrieved from http://www.lifeissues.org/euthanasia/pdf/your_life_your_choices.pdf

Living Trust Network. (2021). Retrieved from https://www.livingtrustnetwork.com/

Mayo Clinic. (2020). Alzheimer's: Dealing with family conflict. Retrieved from https://www.mayoclinic.org/healthy-lifestyle/caregivers/in-depth/art-20047365

National Hospice and Palliative Care Organization. (2020). Retrieved from https://www.nhpco.org/patients-and-caregivers/?pageid=1

National Institute on Aging. (n.d.). Retrieved from https://www.nia.nih.gov/

New York Organ Donor Network. (2014). What organs can be donated? Retrieved from http://www.donatelifeny.org/about-donation/what-can-be-donated/

RBC Wealth Management. (2020). Transferring wealth: Creating a legacy through estate planning. Retrieved from https://www.rbcwm-usa.com/resources/file-687698.pdf

Segal, T. (2019). Questions to ask your estate-planning attorney. Retrieved from https://www.investopedia.com/articles/personal-finance/070815/10-questions-ask-your-estate-planning-attorney.asp

U.S. Government. (2014). Writing a will. Retrieved from http://www.usa.gov/topics/money/personal-finance/wills.shtml

Continue reading to see a selection from another Omega Press title, available now on Amazon.

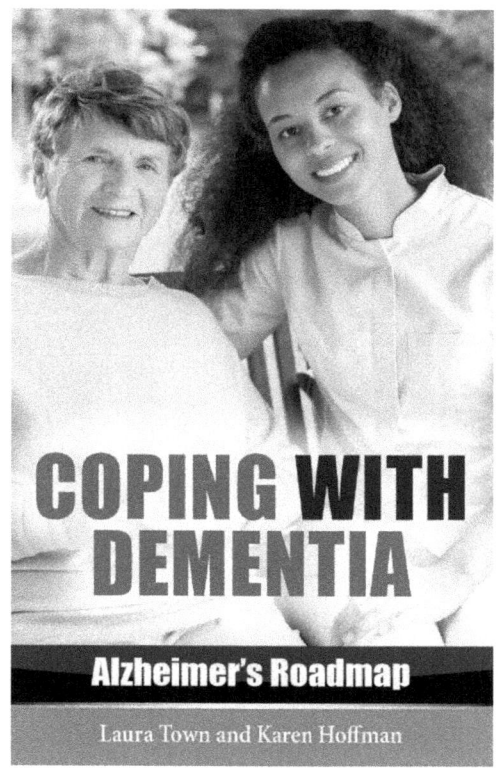

# Coping with Dementia

People, whether they be friends or strangers, will be sympathetic when you tell them that a loved one has dementia. Not knowing how to respond, people will try to find something positive to say about your tragedy—and dementia is tragic. The one comment that bothered me (Laura) the most, although the intention behind it was good, was that at least my father "doesn't know what's happening to him." This is completely false. My dad, in the early and even in the mid stages, knew what was happening. Yes, he couldn't articulate it all the time. Yes, he could not go into detail about the functions of the brain or give a scientific explanation of what was happening. But he knew that he could no longer complete simple tasks. He cried when he could no longer drive. He was enraged when he could not remember the names of his relatives. And he sank into a deep depression when he had to start wearing adult diapers. Even in the late stages when dad was living in a locked dementia unit and before he became nonverbal, my father pointed to adults rocking baby dolls and said to me that he wished he wasn't one of "those people."

Dad's doctor told me that if you've seen one case of Alzheimer's disease, it just means that you've seen one case of Alzheimer's disease, meaning that all cases are different. Perhaps some people slide straight from complete cognition to the late stages of Alzheimer's disease and truly do not have any frustration while being in the throes of the disease, but I have never heard of this.

So people with dementia do know, on a fundamental level, what is happening. That doesn't mean that they know it every day, or even every hour, or become obsessed with their declining health. Dad still had happy moments. He still enjoyed taking walks, listening to music, seeing his grandsons, and eating cupcakes. As long as he was able, I still took him out to restaurants for lunch and dinner or brought him to my house. And although he wasn't particularly religious, he enjoyed visits with the ministers and volunteers who came and read the Bible to him. The challenge is to find what your loved one enjoys and then try to incorporate the enjoyment of it into as many moments of their life as you are able. If you are the one suffering from dementia, then think about what gives you pleasure and find a way to do those things as often as you are able.

When your loved one is diagnosed with Alzheimer's disease or another type of dementia, the emotional effect on the whole family is tremendous. As much as possible, the person with dementia has to come to terms with living with a terminal degenerative disease. They must reckon with a failing memory as well as an increasing reliance on others while also dealing with a society that may feel they have lost their value. Once they enter middle- and later-stage dementia, the disease will begin to affect emotional responses as well as the ability to communicate.

Caregivers, family, and friends of the person with dementia must also process powerful emotions about the news. If your parent, spouse, or other loved one is diagnosed with dementia, you might experience grief over your loved one's loss of memory as well as confusion and stress over practical medical, legal, and financial issues. Your family will likely face some major challenges as you collectively adapt to meet the new needs of the person with dementia. Most significantly, the day-to-day stress of caregiving can take a profound toll on your physical and mental well-being. Being a caregiver affects all parts of your life—personal, professional, and financial—and you may feel that you don't have more than a few minutes to yourself each day. This daily stress can continue for years—sometimes a decade or longer—with serious health implications for you and your family. Studies have found that caregivers' own health problems can be caused or exacerbated by the constant stress of providing care. Studies have also shown that stressed caregivers effectively age faster than people without chronic caregiving responsibilities. According to an American Association of Retired Persons (AARP) report from 2015, 34.2 million Americans provided unpaid care to an adult age 50 or older in the prior 12 months. According to the same report, caregivers spend an average of 24.4 hours a week providing care, with nearly a quarter spending 41 hours or more on care each week, and those caring for a spouse or partner spending 44.6 hours a week. That's an enormous time investment that leaves significantly less time for paid employment and leisure activities. It's easy to see from this how easily caregiving can become all-consuming for the people who provide it.

This book examines the emotional fallout of dementia, and specifically how people with the disease, their caregivers, and their non-caregiver family and friends can cope with that fallout. You'll read about the stages of the disease and how to cope with the common changes at each step. You'll also read about problems that often accompany a terminal chronic illness such as Alzheimer's disease—depression, anxiety, anger, guilt, sleep disturbances, and suicide risk—and how to respond healthily to each of these problems. You'll also get tips and advice for how to support others over the course of dementia: the loved one with the disease, other caregivers, and other family and friends. Although there are different types of dementia including Alzheimer's disease, our checklists should be applicable regardless of the specific diagnosis, and so "dementia" is the term used throughout this book for Alzheimer's disease and other types.

## Emotional Considerations for the Individual with Dementia

Dementia destroys the cognitive function of the individual with the disease. Its effects are catastrophic. The reality is that if you have dementia, you will not only lose the ability to think and remember clearly. You will experience extreme behavioral and emotional changes as the disease progresses, will no longer recognize family members or close friends, and may even develop irrational fears and paranoias. Everyone experiences a loss of function and independence as they age. This is often an emotional struggle. But for people with dementia, these normal changes are compounded in every way and are accompanied by other fundamental changes in how they think, speak, and act.

If you have been diagnosed with dementia, all of this will be painful and overwhelming to confront. This is why the first thing you need to do when you are diagnosed, the only thing you need to do, is allow yourself to experience your emotions. This will be different for every person, but this process is very likely to be similar to the stages of grief as defined by the psychiatrist Elisabeth Kübler-Ross: denial, anger, bargaining, depression, and, finally, acceptance. Give yourself the time and permission to experience and move through these emotions. If you need to feel angry, feel angry. If you need to feel depressed, feel depressed. Try not to lash out at others, but experience all the emotions it's natural to feel at this time. Try to talk to other people about how you feel and try not to isolate yourself, but at the same time, do what you need to do. Don't be ashamed of anything you feel right now. Your emotions are telling you what you need. Listen. There will be a time for understanding and for making important decisions, but that time is not when you are first diagnosed. This time is for you to figure out a way to confront this disease that seems most natural to you.

Once you have experienced the emotions you need to experience, then it is time to seek help to get some of the legal and financial documents you need in place. You won't want to think about this, but it is important to do now while you can still think clearly and make these important decisions for yourself. You can get help with this from your loved ones and learn the basics steps by reading *Long-Term Care Insurance, Power of Attorney, Wealth Management, and Other First Steps*. These first steps come with their own emotional struggles, and it's okay to embrace and experience those emotions, too. You're not alone in this, and whenever you need it, ask for help along the way.

The next two sections examine how to begin understanding the progression of dementia and coping with the diagnosis from the perspective of the individual with the disease. Then the following section turns to the caregiver to suggest ways that caregivers can help with that coping.

## How Dementia Progresses

One thing that may help you if you have been diagnosed with dementia is to learn what the disease is and what it does. Probably the best way to approach understanding dementia is to learn what you should expect as the disease progresses. Although the effects of dementia and how it progresses are different for everyone who has it, generally people with dementia experience a gradual worsening of symptoms over time. In the early stages, memory loss and reduction of ability to function are minor and very gradual, but in the later phases, people with dementia lose the ability to participate in give-and-take conversation and react to stimuli. If you have dementia, activities you used to do easily, such as balancing a checkbook or keeping track of your keys, will become gradually more difficult. The checklist below focuses on the early changes to expect.

*Checklist: Early changes to expect with dementia*

- ☐ Disruptive memory loss, such as forgetting information you learned recently and important dates and events. You may ask for the same information again and again, but you may not remember that you've already asked for it.
- ☐ Difficulty solving problems, such planning an event and keeping track of bills. Working with numbers or following processes with many steps may become especially difficult.
- ☐ Being confused about time and place. You may have trouble remembering what day it is, why

you are where you are and what you were doing, or what is happening right now.

- ☐ Misplacing things, such as not finding car keys where you expect them to be.
- ☐ Difficulty performing familiar work or personal tasks. This may make it challenging or impossible to continue working if you are not retired.
- ☐ Problems with self-expression, such as difficulty organizing thoughts or finding the right words to say what you mean. This may make it difficult for you to follow conversations or to take an active part in them.
- ☐ Impaired judgment that compromises decision making. This may be difficult for you to be aware of, but if you think you've paid for a good or service you haven't received, you notice charges that don't look right to you in your credit card statements, or you receive strange bills, ask for help from your caregivers in understanding what concerns you.
- ☐ Changes in mood and personality, such as depression, anxiety, or sudden and unpredictable irritability and anger. You may become socially withdrawn, even if you are normally very social, and you may lose motivation to complete tasks, especially challenging ones.

# How to Cope if You Have Been Diagnosed with Dementia

If you feel embarrassed by your symptoms and are afraid to talk to others or ask for help, you are not alone. Many people with dementia experience this. However, trying to cover up the symptoms can be very stressful, and eventually it's impossible to cover up the signs. Instead, you should try to integrate changes from the disease into daily life while remaining as active and engaged as possible. If you have been diagnosed, remember to be flexible, fine-tune your approach from day to day, and ask for help. Although some people stigmatize the need to depend on others as weak and parasitic, it is wrong to view relationships this way, especially your relationships with close family and friends. People help one another not just out of a sense of obligation but also to find meaning and purpose in their own lives. If you let other people help you, you can better cope with the disease, and you may also help them cope better with it as well by giving them a way to deal with it. Remember: You and the ones who love and care for you are all in this together.

## *Checklist: How to cope with a diagnosis of dementia*

- ☐ Research dementia and discuss your feelings and findings with loved ones.
- ☐ Involve family and friends in your efforts to learn all you can about dementia.
- ☐ Ask all medical providers to explain medical terms and instructions that you find confusing

or do not remember. Encourage a close family member or friend to assist you in these efforts, helping you take note of anything important for you to know about your diagnosis.

- ☐ Find out what support services are available in your community. Local organizations may offer everything from transportation help to peer counseling.
- ☐ Decide who your primary caregivers should be and, with their help, begin creating and organizing a daily routine for yourself.
- ☐ If you feel overwhelmed with depression, anxiety, and stress following your diagnosis, don't hesitate to seek out a mental health provider. Meeting with a mental health professional early in the course of the disease can help you cope better as the condition worsens. For information on finding a mental health provider, see the Resources at the end of this book.

www.ingramcontent.com/pod-product-compliance
Lightning Source LLC
Chambersburg PA
CBHW061330040426
42444CB00011B/2849